Spanish for Animal Scientists and Food Animal Producers

Spanish for Animal Scientists and Food Animal Producers

Bonnie Frederick and Juan Mosqueda

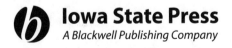

Iowa State Press

A Blackwell Publishing Company

BONNIE FREDERICK, PhD, is a professor of Spanish, Department of Spanish and Latin American Studies, Texas Christian University, Forth Worth.

JUAN MOSQUEDA, MVZ, PhD, is a veterinarian with Centro Nacional de Investigaciones en Parasitología Veterinaria, Jiutipec, Morelos, Mexico.

© 2003 Iowa State Press
A Blackwell Publishing Company
All rights reserved

Iowa State Press
2121 State Avenue, Ames, Iowa 50014

Orders: 1-800-862-6657
Office: 1-515-292-0140
Fax: 1-515-292-3348
Web site: www.iowastatepress.com

∞ Printed on acid-free paper in the United States of America

First edition, 2003

Library of Congress Cataloging-in-Publication Data

Frederick, Bonnie
    Spanish for animal scientists and food animal producers / by Bonnie Frederick and Juan
    Mosqueda.—1st ed.
        p. cm.
    ISBN 0-8138-0267-9 (alk. paper)
    1. Spanish language—Conversation and phrase books (for animal specialists)
I. Mosqueda, Juan. II. Title.

PC4120.A54F74 2003
468.3'421'024636—dc21

                                                                            2003003937

The last digit is the print number: 9   8   7   6   5   4   3   2   1

Contents

Preface

Spanish for Animal Scientists and Food Animal Producers will not make you fluent in Spanish, nor is it intended to do so. Instead, it will teach you how to handle simple, common conversations with Spanish-speaking coworkers. You won't be able to analyze poetry in Spanish, but you will be able to say, "Tell Juan to mend the fence." You won't be able to discuss world politics, but you will be able to say, "The ram isn't eating well. Better call the vet." You will be able to make small talk—"Looks like a storm is coming"—and you'll be able to handle simple courtesies—: "See you tomorrow." You'll learn the vocabulary of feed, tools, and farm buildings, but you won't learn the secret language of grammarians. The grammar presented here is explained in simple ways that avoid jargon, and all the examples are as practical and useful to the animal sciences as possible. For discussing animal illnesses, see the book *Spanish for Veterinarians: A Practical Introduction.* For discussing filling the feed trough or milking the cows, this is the book for you.

The authors would like to thank the faculty and the students of the Animal Sciences Department at Washington State University, Pullman, Washington, for their help and encouragement in creating this book. In particular, we wish to thank the students of the course "Spanish for Animal Sciences" for their many suggestions of terms and phrases to include.

Pronunciation CD

A pronunciation CD accompanies this text and can be found in the pocket inside the back cover. Pronunciation rules, vocabulary, and exercise answers that you will hear are identified by a CD icon (⌀) in the text.

Before listening to the CD, first work out your answers to the exercises and check them with the answer key. Once you have done that, you'll be ready to hear some of the answers spoken by two different native speakers of Spanish. Concentrate on repeating the sounds you hear. For some tracks, you won't need to refer to the book, and so you can work on your pronunciation anywhere you can listen to the CD.

1: Chapter 1, Review of pronunciation rules for vowels and consonants.
2: Chapter 1, Review of rules for the pronounced stress.
3: Chapter 1, Exercises 1, 2, and 3: pronunciation practice.
4: Chapter 2, Vocabulary: animal names, and titles and professions.
5: Chapter 2, Exercises 1, 2, and 3: articles and plurals.
6: Chapter 3, Exercises 1, 2, and 3: adjectives.
7: Chapter 3, Exercises 5, 6, 7, and 8: adjectives of distance and possession.
8: Chapter 3, Vocabulary: buildings and grounds.
9: Chapter 4, Exercise 2: matching verbs with their subjects.

Spanish for
Animal Scientists
and Food Animal
Producers

CHAPTER 1

Pronunciation

I'm going to let you in on the language teachers' Great Secret: really good pronunciation lets you fudge the grammar and vocabulary. There's a corollary to this secret, which is that perfect grammar won't make up for bad pronunciation. Don't take this secret as permission to ignore grammar, but do take it as good advice to work hard on pronunciation.

Fortunately, English-speaking students can breathe a sigh of relief: Spanish is simple, regular, and logical in its pronunciation. Best of all, written Spanish faithfully reflects its pronunciation. Thank goodness it's not like English! Think of the poor students of English who have to wrestle with letters that don't represent sounds. For example, "tough," "though," "through," and "thought" all have the letters *ough,* but they are pronounced in four different ways. Spanish isn't like that. It's a "superior" language in this respect!

There are three general characteristics of Spanish pronunciation that make it different from English pronunciation:

1. The vowels are more important than the consonants. This is the opposite of English, which is a consonant-dominant language. So when you begin to pronounce Spanish, you need to give the vowels a lot more attention than you're accustomed to giving them. Pronounce them clearly; don't swallow them or slide over them. No mumbling over vowels!

2. Each sound is maintained for only one beat; you shouldn't hold on to it: *a* not *aaa.* English, especially the English of the southern United States, hangs on to sounds, stretching them out like a kid stringing out bubble gum. Don't do this in Spanish. Instead, make your sounds clipped and compressed.

3. There is only one stressed syllable per word. English has both major and minor stresses in a word, making it sound singsongy to Spanish speakers. In Spanish, there are three simple rules for stresses, and only one stress occurs per word, so it's practically stress free to learn!

Now that you're prepared with the general characteristics, let's look at the particular ones.

NOTE

The following pronunciation guidelines are for Latin American Spanish, with preference given to Mexican pronunciation.

Vowel Sounds

English speakers should first focus on the vowels:

a as in f<u>a</u>ther, <u>o</u>tter, m<u>o</u>dern
e as in <u>a</u>ble, <u>ei</u>ght, p<u>ai</u>nt
i as in <u>ea</u>sy, <u>ea</u>t, mach<u>i</u>ne
o as in b<u>oa</u>t, r<u>o</u>pe, <u>O</u>K
u as in l<u>oo</u>p, m<u>oo</u>, d<u>u</u>de

Now try out these words, saying them out loud slowly, paying great attention to the vowels (don't worry about the other sounds or the words' meanings yet):

alimento
agua

ensilaje
establo
industria
infertilidad
ollar
ombligo
uso
úlcera

Generally speaking, the vowels are more important in Spanish than in English, so you should practice them a lot!

Consonant Sounds _____

The consonants are similar to those in English, with these exceptions:

- *d* — Very soft; it's similar to "<u>th</u>ese". When the *d* occurs between two vowels, it might even disappear in rapid speech; *hablado* can become *hablao* in some varieties of Spanish. Some practice words: *aditivo, ganadero, producción.*
- *h* — Silent. No matter how tempting it is, don't pronounce it. Practice: *heces, hongo, hato.*
- *j* — Pronounced like the English "<u>h</u>appy." Practice: *Juan, granja, manejo.*
- *ll* — Pronounced like the English "<u>y</u>ahoo", except in some dialects (especially in Argentina), in which case it's pronounced like "<u>J</u>ell-o." Try both ways: *llama, semilla, ampolla.*
- *ñ* — Like "can<u>y</u>on". Indeed, the word in Spanish is *cañón.* Try these: *español, ordeñar, rebaño.*
- *qu* — Like "<u>k</u>ick", not "quick"; it doesn't have the *w* sound as in English. Practice: *quijada, tanque, equipo.*
- *r* — Inside a word there is a little flip of the tongue as in the English words "ba<u>tt</u>er," "bi<u>tt</u>er," or "bu<u>tt</u>er." Practice

the English example words first, then while your tongue is loosened up, try: *minerales, litro, esteroide.*

- *rr* — To pronounce *rr* or *r* at the beginning of a word, you must first practice purring like a cat or making a car's revving-up sound. The sound should be in your tongue (flapping like a flag in the wind) and not in your throat (no hacking please). First rev up or purr, then practice these words: *corral, rumen, becerro, raza.*

- *v* — Pronounced like "<u>b</u>ed." It is common for uneducated people to switch the *b* and the *v* in their spelling. For example, it is not unusual to see *javón* (soap) instead of the correct form, *jabón.* Practice: *vacuna, bovino, ave.*

- *x* — Usually pronounced as in English; here is *x* in its usual *ks* form: *toxina, examen, sexo.* But in certain words with origin in indigenous languages, *x* is more like the Spanish *j.* Try these *j* sound words: *México, Oaxaca.*

- *z* — Pronounced like *s* in Latin America: *maíz, Martínez, pezón.*

Finally, *c* and *g* can be hard or soft, depending on what follows the letter:

- *c* — Hard like *k* when it is followed by *a, o,* or *u.* Practice: *calor, consumo, campo.* But it is soft like *s* when it is followed by *i* or *e.* Try: *ciencia, celo, comercial.*

- *g* — Like "gargle" when it's followed by *a, o,* or *u.* Practice: *ganado, gota, Guzmán.* Followed by *e* or *i,* the *g* becomes softened into a "<u>h</u>ello" sound: *genética, Gilberto, gestación.*

✐ Where Does the Stress Go?

There are three rules for stress pronunciation.

1. If a word ends in a vowel, an *s,* or an *n,* then the stress is on the next-to-the-last syllable: <u>son</u>da, <u>co</u>bre, <u>cli</u>ma, <u>le</u>che, <u>se</u>men, <u>es</u>tro, <u>va</u>cas.

2. If a word ends in a consonant except an *s* or an *n,* the
   stress is on the last syllable: *ani̱mal, tropi̱cal, pe̱sar, salu̱d,
   fecundi̱dad, pie̱l.*
3. If a word doesn't follow rule 1 or rule 2, then there's a written
   accent mark: *bisturi̱, o̱vulo, ce̱lula, vi̱scera, difi̱cil.*

Do you want to hear these sounds as pronounced by native speakers of
Spanish? Check out the CD packaged in this book. And then practice,
practice, practice!

EXERCISE 1-1

Referring to the stress rules above, first underline the syllable in the
words below that should be stressed, then pronounce the words, paying
particular attention to the vowels. Then listen to the CD and repeat
the words after the native speakers.

1. alfalfa
2. buche
3. corral
4. celo
5. desinfectar
6. ensilaje
7. fiebre
8. garrapata
9. Geraldo
10. heno
11. inseminar
12. joroba
13. leche
14. mastitis
15. novillo
16. oveja
17. pasto
18. quiste
19. rumen
20. sangre

21. ternero
22. ubre
23. vaquilla
24. yodo
25. zanahoria

EXERCISE 1-2

These words do not follow the stress rules, so they have a written accent mark. Try pronouncing the words on your own, then listen to the CD and repeat the words after the native speakers.

1. láctea
2. gestación
3. inglés
4. estrés
5. número
6. corazón
7. vesícula
8. marrón
9. cólera
10. dósis
11. estómago
12. fértil
13. glándula
14. tórax
15. González

EXERCISE 1-3

The following words look like English, but they're not. Say them with Spanish pronunciation:

1. rancho
2. normal
3. teléfono
4. semen

5. animal
6. cliente
7. medicina
8. vitamina
9. fundamental
10. doctor
11. hospital
12. diarrea
13. virus
14. pie
15. mastitis
16. pus
17. natural
18. color
19. genética
20. dieta
21. anemia
22. cereal
23. control
24. grave
25. gasolina

STUDY NOTE

Language is a subject in which practice really does make perfect. For example, going once through the exercises above is not enough; you should practice them out loud often. Come back to this chapter while you're studying the following chapters. Take the CD with you as you drive, and use that time for pronunciation practice. At home, if you have a tape recorder, record your second effort (the first time through is for warming up). Listen to how you pronounce the vowels and where you're putting the stress. Compare your efforts with the pronunciation of the native speakers on the CD. Don't be hard on yourself—these are new sounds, and it will take a while to get used to them. Also, the muscles in your mouth have to learn new movements. You can tell you're making progress if your mouth muscles are a little sore. "No pain, no gain!" So be patient, and practice a lot.

The Mistakes We Make in Each Other's Language ⎯

In Spanish, *sp, sc,* and *st* cannot start a word, so *e* is put in front of those sounds. A Spanish speaker will tend to pronounce the English words "special" as "especial"; "school" as "eschool"; and "state" as "estate." Also, Spanish speakers tend to slight English consonants, because consonants are dominated by vowels in Spanish. As a result, English words such as "good," "like," or "hamburger" tend to come out as "goo," "li," and "amburer." Don't panic the first time you hear a Spanish speaker struggling with difficult English pronunciation; with practice, you'll begin to discern the speaker's words, and soon you won't even notice the differences.

Meanwhile, English speakers tend to slight Spanish vowels and give too much attention to the consonants. Plus, they tend to hold on to the syllables too long. As a result, *México* becomes *Meeexcoo*; *español* becomes *espñolll;* and *ciudad* becomes *suuddaadd.* And many English speakers simply give up on the *r* and *rr.* It's true that those sounds can be hard at first, because English speakers haven't exercised the mouth and tongue muscles needed for a rolled *r.* They need mouth aerobics! But flabby-*r* English speakers shouldn't despair—good pronunciation is achievable and is well worth the effort.

CULTURAL NOTE: NAMES

In Spanish-heritage cultures, a person's name reflects both the father's and the mother's names. For example, take my friend's name: Manuel Gutiérrez Marín. *Manuel* is his first name (in Spanish, *nombre de pila,* or "baptismal font name") and *Gutiérrez Marín* is his last name (*apellido* in Spanish).

Gutiérrez is the first part of his father's last name, and
Marín is the first part of his mother's maiden name.
My friend Manuel married Julia Flores Vásquez. *Flores*
is her father's last name, and *Vásquez* is her mother's
maiden name.

Manuel and Julia had a son, Matías. What is his last name?
Answer: Gutiérrez Flores.

Many people just use their father's name (the "patronymic")
for informal occasions, and reserve their full name (with
their mother's maiden name, the "matronymic") for formal
occasions. So, Manuel can be Manuel Gutiérrez if he chooses,
and Julia can be Julia Flores.

Traditionally, women do not change their names after
marriage. They can, if they so desire, indicate their married
status by adding *de* and their husband's name. For example,
Manuel's wife Julia can write her name like this: *Julia Flores
Vásquez de Gutiérrez.* Or she can be *Julia Flores de Gutiérrez.*
An important Peruvian author was Clorinda Matto de
Turner. What was her husband's last name? Answer: Turner.

Names are alphabetized under the patronymic. So, the
Nobel Prize–winning author Gabriel García Márquez should
be alphabetized under *García.*

In the United States it's not easy to keep Hispanic or
Latino culture alive under the pressure of Anglo-American
culture, so many people hyphenate their names to keep
them from being split up or misunderstood. That's why my
friend Marielena Pérez Cantú writes her name as Marielena
Pérez-Cantú when she's away from her native Puerto Rico.

The *ez* at the end of many Spanish names means "son
of," just as Johnson means "son of John," Fitzpatrick means
"son of Patrick," and MacDonald means "son of Donald."
So *Rodríguez* is literally "son of Rodrigo," *González* "son of
Gonzalo," and *Martínez* "son of Martín."

An interesting aside about Hispanic names: the U.S. Census
Bureau, 2000, reports that the most common last name in

the United States, Smith, is already being outnumbered in some areas of the country by the most common Hispanic last name, García. García is predicted to become the most common last name in the whole country by the middle of the twenty-first century. Look at your town's phone book to see if this trend is apparent where you live.

CHAPTER 2

Nouns and Articles

What are nouns? They are people, places, and things; often they have "the" in front of them. Here are some nouns: the chair, the building, the cow, the ranch, Mom. What are articles? The direct article is "the." The indirect articles are "a" and "an."

In Spanish, nouns have gender; they are either masculine or feminine. A long time ago, English used to have gendered nouns. If you've read *Beowulf* or Chaucer's *Canterbury Tales* in their original English (as I'm sure you do in your spare time), you've seen examples. These days, there are only a few gendered nouns left in English, such as ships, which are often referred to with feminine pronouns: "the ship, she is sinking."

But in Spanish, all nouns are either masculine or feminine: books are masculine; machines are feminine; paper is masculine; tables are feminine. The masculine form of "the" is *el*, and the feminine form of "the" is *la*: *el libro* [the book], *la máquina* [the machine], *el papel* [the paper], *la mesa* [the table].

Guidelines for Determining a Noun's Gender _____

• Feminine nouns often end in *a*: *la yegua, la cabra, la pezuña, la computadora.*

- Masculine nouns often end in *o: el cerdo, el ordeño, el establo, el ganado.* Exception: *la mano.*
- Words that end in *itis, osis, ción, sión, dad, tad, tud, ía, ie,* or *umbre* are usually feminine: *la mastitis, la brucelosis, la reproducción, la lesión, la calidad, la dificultad, la multitud, la lechería, la intemperie, la cumbre.*
- Just to keep things lively, Spanish absorbed a lot of Greek words. In Greek, a word ending in *a* is usually masculine. That's why "it's Greek to me": *el problema, el sistema, el programa, el diafragma, el día.* Notice that most, though not all, of these words end in *ema.*
- Words that end in *ón* (note: not *ción* or *sión*; see above) are usually masculine: *el corazón, el embrión, el avión, el sillón.*
- There often are pairs of words showing the actual gender of a person or animal: *la veterinaria, el veterinario; la coneja, el conejo; la cerda, el cerdo; la dueña, el dueño; la obrera, el obrero.*
- If two words are combined to make one new word, the new word is masculine. For example, *para* [stop] + *brisas* [winds] = *el parabrisas* [windshield]. More examples: *el paraguas* [umbrella], *el pasaporte* [passport], *el tranvía* [tram], *el saltamontes* [grasshopper], *el montacargas* [forklift].
- Beyond these guidelines, you simply have to learn the noun's gender when you learn the noun. As you study vocabulary, always learn the word with its *el* or *la*. Notice, for example, that the following words both end in *e* but differ in gender: *la sangre, el forraje.*

Articles and Plurals

The definite article, "the" in English, is *la* or *el*, as we saw previously. The indefinite articles, "a" or "an" in English, are *una* (feminine) or *un* (masculine):

la semilla [the seed], *una semilla* [a seed]
el rancho [the ranch], *un rancho* [a ranch]
la raza [the breed], *una raza* [a breed]
el rebaño [the flock of sheep or goats], *un rebaño* [a flock of
   sheep or goats]

An *s* at the end of the noun makes it plural. *El* becomes *los, la* becomes
las, un becomes *unos,* and *una* becomes *unas:*

las semillas [the seeds], *unas semillas* [some seeds]
los ranchos [the ranches], *unos ranchos* [some ranches]
las razas [the breeds], *unas razas* [some breeds]
los rebaños [the flocks of sheep or goats], *unos rebaños* [some
   flocks of sheep or goats]

If a word ends in a consonant, add *es* instead of *s:*

el corral [the corral], *los corrales* [the corrals]
la dificultad [the difficulty], *las dificultades* [the difficulties]
una piel [a hide, skin], *unas pieles* [some hides, skins]
un sifón [a syphon], *unos sifones* [some syphons]

✐ Animal Names

English	male	female	offspring	collective form, such as "herd" or "flock"
cattle, cows	el toro	la vaca	la ternera el ternero	el ganado el hato
swine	el cerdo	la cerda	la lechona el lechón	la piara
sheep	el carnero	la oveja	la cordera el cabrito	el rebaño

(continues)

(continued)

English	male	female	offspring	collective form, such as "herd" or "flock"
goats	el macho cabrío *or* la cabra macho*	la cabra	la cabrita el cabrito	el rebaño
chickens	el gallo	la gallina	la pollita el pollito	la parvada
turkeys	el pavo *or* el guajolote**	la pava	el pavito la pavita	la pavada
ducks	el pato	la pata	la patita el patito	la bandada
rabbits	el conejo	la coneja	la conejita el conejito	los conejos

*   The official word for a male goat has become a vulgarity in Spanish, so these socially acceptable substitutes are used instead.

** In Mexico, where turkeys are native, the Aztec word for "turkey" was guajolote, and that term is still used today. In some rural areas of Mexico, they use the term cócono. Processed turkey meat, though, is called pavo, as is the roasted version served on holidays. English speakers should say pavo but be able to recognize guajolote if they hear it. By the way, a pavo real or "royal turkey" is the term for a peacock.

✐ Special Vocabulary: Titles and Professions _____

agent	el agente, la agenta
boss	el jefe, la jefa
buyer	el comprador, la compradora
cowboy, cowgirl	el vaquero, la vaquera

foreman	el mayordomo, la mayordomo; el capataz, la capataz
friend	el amigo, la amiga
herder	el pastor, la pastora
inspector	el inspector, la inspectora
milker	el ordeñador, la ordeñadora
neighbor	el vecino, la vecina
nutritionist	el nutriólogo, la nutrióloga
owner	el dueño, la dueña
representative	el representante, la representante
seller	el vendedor, la vendedora
veterinarian	el veterinario, la veterinaria
worker	el obrero, la obrera

EXERCISE 2-1

What is the gender of the following nouns? They follow the guidelines at the beginning of this chapter. Write *el* or *la* in front of the word to show its gender. Example: *toro = el toro*. After you have written your answers, either in this book or on a scratch sheet of paper, check your answers in the answer key at the back of the book. But don't look at the answer key before you do the exercise! (In this and the following exercises in this chapter, don't worry about the meaning of the words yet.)

1. torta
2. alimento
3. estómago
4. enfermedad
5. camión
6. reproducción
7. alfalfa
8. ensilaje
9. influenza
10. problema
11. gestación

12. hocico
13. escroto
14. bronquitis
15. separador

EXERCISE 2-2

Change the definite article to the indefinite article. Example: *el toro* = *un toro.*

1. el cerdo
2. la epidemia
3. el animal
4. el cordero
5. la garrapata
6. la piara
7. el sistema
8. la granja
9. el baño
10. la incubadora

EXERCISE 2-3

Change the following nouns to their plural form. Example: *el toro = los toros, un toro = unos toros.*

1. la ubre
2. el parto
3. una pocilga
4. un freno
5. el biberón
6. un vaquero
7. la esquiladora
8. una gallina
9. el tractor
10. la jaula
11. una pala

12. un mineral
13. el trinchete
14. la enzima
15. un ingrediente

STUDY NOTE: LEARNING VOCABULARY

You're probably asking yourself, "How the heck am I going to learn all these words?" Don't panic—instead, make flash cards. Flash cards are simple, efficient, portable, and reviewable. In other words, they're about the best way for you to learn new words and retain them.

Make your flash cards by cutting up some paper into pieces about the size of a credit card. Now write the Spanish word on one side (don't forget to include the *el* or the *la!*) and its English equivalent on the other side. Just making the cards is a good study technique; don't ever buy commercial flash cards, because they can't provide you with this initial reinforcement.

Now, look at the Spanish side of the cards. Say the Spanish word out loud, and guess what the English equivalent is. If you get it right, put that card in one stack, and if you get it wrong, put the card in another stack. After going through all the cards, return to the stack of cards you guessed wrong on, and keep reviewing them until you get them right.

Next, turn the cards over. Look at the English side, and guess what the Spanish equivalent is. Make two stacks as you did before.

Tuck your flash cards into your pocket, and practice with them at idle moments. Waiting for an appointment with the doctor, for example, is an excellent opportunity to run through your flash cards. Stick them on the bathroom mirror so that you can look at them as you shave or put on makeup in the morning. Practicing with a friend or spouse is a good technique too. Keep your old flash cards in a shoe box so that you can review them from time to time.

How many words can you learn in a week? If you mean learn *and retain,* probably about five to eight new words a day. Don't try to memorize the whole dictionary at once. Torturing yourself with long lists of vocabulary will take all the fun out of learning, and besides, it's unlikely you'll retain the vocabulary under those circumstances. It's much more productive to assign yourself to learn about five to eight new words a day, as well as reviewing about the same number of words you've learned previously. Take Saturday and Sunday off.

Where should you begin? Start your vocabulary project by making flash cards for the animal names and titles listed in this chapter. The following chapters will identify the words you should learn under the heading "Special Vocabulary."

CULTURAL NOTE: NICKNAMES

Just as the English names "James" and "Patricia" become "Jim" and "Patty" among friends, many Spanish names have nicknames, that is, affectionate forms used by friends and family. Here are some common nicknames:

Francisco	Paco
María	Maruca
Ignacio	Nacho
Guadalupe	Lupe
Jesús	Chuy; in the United States, Jessie
Dolores	Lola
Antonio	Toño
Antonia	Toñita
José	Pepe
Josefina	Pepita; in the United States, Josie

Vicente	Chente
Enrique	Quique
Enriqueta	Queta
Alfonso	Poncho
Graciela	Chela
Eduardo	Lalo

Another way to make an affectionate name is to add *ito* or *ita* to the end. For example, *Juan* [John] and *Juana* [Jane] can become *Juanito* [Johnny] and *Juanita* [Janie]. Children often have this done to their names; for instance, little Pedro, aged three, becomes *Pedrito* and little Guadalupe becomes *Lupita*.

Other nicknames aren't based on the person's official name but instead on personality or looks. A very skinny person could become *Flaco* or *Flaca,* for example. Such nicknames aren't as accepted in English-speaking countries as they are in Spanish-speaking ones. Therefore, it may surprise you that although *Gordito* or *Gordita* is literally "fatty," it actually has the emotional content of "deary" or "honey." The lullaby *"Duerme, duerme, negrito"* [Sleep, sleep little Black baby] is the emotional equivalent of "Sleep, sleep little sweetheart." And calling one's father *Viejo* [old man] is affectionate, not disrespectful, probably because being old in Hispanic culture is not a negative condition.

If you are around Spanish speakers a lot, you will hear nicknames. Should you use them yourself? Generally speaking, if people introduce themselves with their nicknames, then they are inviting you to use them too; but if a person introduces himself or herself with his or her official name, then you should use that name.

CHAPTER 3

Adjectives

What are adjectives? They are words that describe nouns, giving us more information. For example, "the cow" doesn't include much information by itself. But "the little, one-eyed, feisty cow" gives enough information so that we know which one she is. In Spanish, the adjective matches the noun in gender and number. That is, if the noun is singular and feminine, the adjective describing it is also singular and feminine. If the noun is masculine and plural, so is its adjective.

For example, let's take the color "white" and add it to some nouns: *la vaca blanca* [the white cow]; *el cerdo blanco* [the white boar]; *las ovejas blancas* [the white ewes]; *los camiones blancos* [the white trucks]. Notice that the idea of "white" changes form to always reflect the noun it is describing.

Unlike English, Spanish usually puts its adjectives after the noun, not before it: don't say, *la blanca vaca;* say, *la vaca blanca.* (Exceptions to this rule are discussed a little further on.)

Some Common Adjectives

big	grande
black	negro, negra
brown	pardo, parda

calm, tame	manso, mansa
frisky, spirited	fogoso, fogosa
lame, limping	cojo, coja
long (in length)	largo, larga
new	nuevo, nueva
newborn	recién nacido, recién nacida
old	viejo, vieja
pregnant	preñada
red	rojo, roja
short (in length)	corto, corta
small	pequeño, pequeña; chico, chica
white	blanco, blanca

EXERCISE 3-1

Change the following phrases to Spanish. For example, change "a black cow" to *una vaca negra.*

1. the white sow
2. a new hen
3. the newborn calf (m.)
4. the brown kid (f.)
5. an old bull
6. the pregnant ewe
7. a big boar
8. the black rooster
9. the small ram
10. a red cow

EXERCISE 3-2

Now change the phrases to their plural form. For example, change "some black cows" to *unas vacas negras.*

1. the white sows
2. some new hens
3. the newborn calves (m.)

4. the brown kids (f.)
5. some old bulls
6. the pregnant ewes
7. some big boars
8. the black roosters
9. the small rams
10. some red cows

Numbers and Number Words

Which adjectives go before the noun, not after it? You already know one answer to this question: the articles go in front. Another answer? Numbers go in front. Numbers don't show gender, with the exception of the number words *mucho* [many] and *poco* [few].

1	uno, una, un. (*Un* is used in front of the noun: *un libro* [one book]. *Uno* is used alone: How many calves are left in the truck? *Uno* [one])
2	dos
3	tres
4	cuatro
5	cinco
6	seis
7	siete
8	ocho
9	nueve
10	diez
11	once
12	doce
13	trece
14	catorce
15	quince
16	dieciséis
17	diecisiete
18	dieciocho
19	diecinueve

20	veinte
29	veintinueve
30	treinta
38	treinta y ocho
40	cuarenta
47	cuarenta y siete
50	cincuenta
56	cincuenta y seis
60	sesenta
65	sesenta y cinco
70	setenta
74	setenta y cuatro
80	ochenta
83	ochenta y tres
90	noventa
92	noventa y dos
100	ciento (If it's placed in front of a noun, it becomes just *cien*.)
120	ciento veinte
200	doscientos, doscientas
300	trescientos, trescientas
400	cuatrocientos, cuatrocientas
500	quinientos, quinientas
600	seiscientos, seiscientas
700	setecientos, setecientas
800	ochocientos, ochocientas
900	novecientos, novecientas
1,000	mil
1,865	mil ochocientos sesenta y cinco

mucho heno [a lot of hay], *mucha leche* [a lot of milk], *muchos corderos* [many lambs], *muchas gallinas* [many hens]

poco heno [not a lot of hay], *poca leche* [not much milk], *pocos corderos* [few lambs, not many lambs], *pocas gallinas* [few hens, not many hens]

EXERCISE 3-3

Change the following phrases to Spanish. For example, change "16 lambs" to *dieciséis corderos.*

1. 6 calves
2. few cows
3. many sheep
4. 182 chicks
5. 17 lambs
6. 12 goats (f.)
7. 24 feeder pigs
8. lots of hens
9. 15 bulls
10. 100 pigs

EXERCISE 3-4

Now add the adjective *nuevo* to the phrases above. For example, change "16 new lambs" to *dieciséis corderos nuevos.*

1. 6 new calves
2. few new cows
3. many new sheep
4. 182 new chicks
5. 17 new lambs
6. 12 new goats (f.)
7. 24 new feeder pigs
8. lots of new hens
9. 15 new bulls
10. 100 new pigs

Distance Adjectives

One other kind of adjective goes before the noun rather than behind it, and that is what we call the "distance adjective," because it shows how far the object is from the speaker. For example, something near to the speaker is "this milking machine," one a little further away is "that milking machine," and one that is distant is "that milking machine over there." These distance adjectives in Spanish show gender and number:

this milking machine	esta ordeñadora
these milking machines	estas ordeñadoras
this filter	este filtro
these filters	estos filtros
that milking machine	esa ordeñadora
those milking machines	esas ordeñadoras
that filter	ese filtro
those filters	esos filtros
that milking machine way over there	aquella ordeñadora
those milking machines way over there	aquellas ordeñadoras
that filter way over there	aquel filtro
those filters way over there	aquellos filtros

EXERCISE 3-5

Change the following phrases to Spanish. For example, change "this black cow" to *esta vaca negra*.

1. this white sow
2. that new hen
3. that newborn calf
4. the brown kid (f.) over there
5. that old bull
6. this pregnant ewe
7. that big boar way over there
8. this black rooster

9. that small ram
10. that red cow over there

Now change the phrases to their plural form. For example, change "these black cows" to *estas vacas negras.*

1. these white sows
2. those new hens
3. those newborn calves
4. those brown kids (f.) over there
5. those old bulls
6. these pregnant ewes
7. those big boars way over there
8. these black roosters
9. those small rams
10. those red cows over there

Possessive Adjectives

Okay, just one more group of adjectives that go in front of the noun, and then you can go back to the general rule that adjectives go after the noun. This group is the possessive adjectives. No, they're not clingy and whiny; they indicate that something belongs to someone. They all can be singular or plural, and one can show the masculine or feminine form. Here they are:

my = *mi,* as in *mi auto* [my car] and *mis autos* [my cars]

your (informal) = *tu,* as in *tu auto* [your car] and *tus autos* [your cars]

his, her, your (formal) = *su,* as in *su auto* [his car, her car, your car] and *sus autos* [his cars, her cars, your cars]

our = *nuestro,* as in *nuestro auto* [our car], *nuestros autos* [our cars], *nuestra casa* [our house], *nuestras casas* [our houses]

their, you guys', ya'll's, your (plural) = *su,* as in *su auto* [their
car, you guys' car], *sus autos* [their cars, you guys' cars]

How can you tell if *su* is talking about his, her, your, or their car? By
the context. If you've been talking about Susana, then you know that
su means "her," but if you've been talking about Susana and Michael,
then you know that *su* means "their." When you're in doubt about
whether someone will know whose possession or attribute you're talking
about, use *de: el auto de Susana* = "Susana's car"; *el auto de Susana y
Miguel* = "Susana and Michael's car."

To sum up: all adjectives are positioned behind the noun, except
articles, numbers, distances, and possessives. These last four groups
are positioned *before* the noun.

EXERCISE 3-7

Change the following phrases to Spanish, using the special vocabulary
below and the possessives. Example: "their house" = *su casa.*

1. my dairy
2. his farm
3. our gate
4. her fence
5. your (formal) water tank
6. their ranch
7. our road

EXERCISE 3-8

Now change the phrase to its plural form. Example: "their houses" =
sus casas.

1. my dairies
2. his farms
3. our gates
4. her fences

5. your (formal) water tanks
6. their ranches
7. our roads

✐ Special Vocabulary: Buildings and Grounds ————

Do you need to know this whole list? Probably not. Just learn the words for the sites on your property. For example, if you don't raise chickens, you can skip *el gallinero*.

cattle ranch	el rancho ganadero
dairy farm	la granja lechera
farm	la granja, la finca
hog farm	la granja porcícola
poultry farm	la granja avícola
ranch	el rancho
sheep ranch	el rancho ovejero
barn; granary	el granero
commodity barn	el almacén
driveway	el camino de entrada
garage	el garaje
(for larger vehicles)	el esta cionamiento
garden	el jardín
gas pump	la bomba de gasolina
henhouse, chicken coop	el gallinero
house	la casa
orchard (large)	la huerta
(small, for a single family)	el huerto
road	el camino
stable; cowshed; barn for animals	el establo
sty, pigsty	la pocilga, el chiquero
water tank	el tanque de agua
workshop	el taller

grain elevator	el almacén de granos, el silo con elevador
hayloft	el henil
haystack	el pajar
milking shed	el local de ordeño
milk-processing building, milk sales building	la lechería
silo	el silo
bin	la caja
box stall	el cubículo
feed trough, feed bunk, feeder	el comedero
grain bin	el granero
grain storage, grain elevator	el almacén de grano
passageway	el corredor, el pasillo
stall	el pesebre
watering trough, drinker	el bebedero
barbed wire	el alambre de púas
electrified fence	la cerca eléctrica
fence	la cerca
fence post	el poste
gate, door	la puerta
wire mesh	la tela metálica
barnyard; pen; corral	el corral
chute	la rampa, la manga
holding pen	el corral contenedor
loading chute	la rampa de embarque
runway, lane	la línea, el pasillo
sorting chute	la manga separadora
sorting pen	el corral separador
squeeze chute	la presa, la trampa
creek	el arroyo
irrigation ditch	la acequia

manure pile	el estercolero
pasture	el pastizal, el pasto, el campo, la pastura
pond	la charca
river	el río

Meeting People

When you meet someone, you have the chance to use your Spanish to good effect, even if your pronunciation isn't perfect and you don't know the whole language, because there are established rituals for introductions that you can learn and use quickly. These rituals consist of customs and polite phrases. The customs include shaking hands at the beginning *and* the end of the introduction, standing a little closer than you probably are accustomed to (see chapter 6 for more details), and not squeezing hard when you shake hands. Here are some polite phrases:

Buenos días. = Good morning.

Buenas tardes. = Good afternoon. (Note: Among Latinos, afternoon goes on until about 7 p.m.)

Me llamo.... = My name is _____. (Literally, "I call myself ....")

Este es mi hijo, ... = This is my son, ... (For other family members, see chapter 12.)

Mucho gusto. = Pleased to meet you.

Bienvenido. = Welcome.

Bienvenido a Omaha. = Welcome to Omaha.

CHAPTER 4

Regular Verbs

What is a verb? It's the word that shows action. Without a verb, the cow can't do anything. With a verb, the cow grazes, the cow moos, the cow chews, the cow breaks the fence, the cow swishes its tail, or the cow kicks the milking machine.

In its raw form, a verb is called an infinitive (I like to think that's because the possibilities are infinite.) In this raw form, the verb ends in either *ar, er,* or *ir.* This infinitive ending has the idea of "to": *hablar* [to speak], *comprar* [to buy], *vivir* [to live], *añadir* [to add], *vender* [to sell], *depender* [to depend].

The verbs change according to who is doing the action. You can see this in English too: "I go, she goes." The verb very specifically indicates who is carrying out the action. Here are the possible actors:

- *Yo,* "I," is indicated in the verb by breaking off the infinitive ending (*ar, ir, er*) and adding *o:*

hablar [to speak] = *yo hablo* [I speak]
vender [to sell] = *vendo* [I sell]
vivir [to live] = *vivo* [I live]

- *Nosotros,* "we," is indicated in the verb by breaking off the infinitive ending and adding *amos, emos, imos:*

hablar = *hablamos* [we speak]
vender = *vendemos* [we sell]
vivir = *vivimos* [we live]

- *Ella, él, usted* ["she," "he," and "you" in its formal sense]
  are indicated in the verb by breaking off the infinitive
  ending and adding *a, e, e:*

hablar = *habla* [she, he speaks; you speak]
vender = *vende* [she, he sells; you sell]
vivir = *vive* [she, he lives; you live]

- *Ellas, ellos, ustedes* [they, ya'll or you guys] are indicated in
  the verb by breaking off the infinitive ending and adding
  an, en, en:

hablar = *hablan* [they speak, ya'll speak]
vender = *venden* [they sell, you guys sell]
vivir = *viven* [they live, ya'll live]

- *Tú* is the form of "you" that is used only to address family,
  good friends, children, animals. You wouldn't use this form
  in a professional setting; in that situation, you'll use *usted.*
  Tú is indicated in the verb by breaking off the infinitive
  and adding *as, es, es:*

hablar = *hablas* [you speak]
vender = *vendes* [you sell]
vivir = *vives* [you live]

It is customary to run a verb through its paces by putting it in a chart
like this, with the singulars in one column and the plurals in another:

Hablar [to speak]

yo hablo	nosotros hablamos
tú hablas	
él, ella, usted habla	ellos, ellas, ustedes hablan

Vender [to sell]

vendo	vendemos
vendes	
vende	venden

Vivir [to live]

vivo	vivimos
vives	
vive	viven

Or, you can list the conjugation (the forms) with the singulars first and the plurals second:

> *hablar = hablo, hablas, habla, hablamos, hablan*
> *vender = vendo, vendes, vende, vendemos, venden*
> *vivir = vivo, vives, vive, vivimos, viven*

In the answer key at the back of this book, the verbs are listed like this, in order to save space. Should you make charts or lists? The answer is whatever helps you learn, according to your own style.

Notice two things about the verbs:

- In Spanish, there's no "it speaks." All things are masculine or feminine in Spanish, so the equivalent in Spanish is "he speaks" or "she speaks." Animals are not "it"; they are "he" or "she": *la vaca camina* = "the cow walks," "she walks."
- Spanish verbs are so specific about who is doing the action that you don't have to repeat the actor. For example, *hablo* can only be "I speak"; it can't be anything else, so you don't have to say *yo hablo*. The exception to this observation is that it is considered courteous to use *usted*: *usted habla*.

Now notice this about English: "I go" can become "I do go," especially when the sentence is a question ("Do you go?") or negative ("I do not go"). The Spanish verbs include this idea in the one simple form *voy* [I go, I do go], *vas* [you go, you do go], *va* [she goes, she does go], and so on.

EXERCISE 4-1

On a scratch sheet of paper, conjugate the following verbs, that is, put them in a chart like the ones above. For the first half of the list, include the subject or actor (as in the *hablar* chart above) until you feel comfortable with the connection between the subject and the verb endings. After that, just conjugate the verbs without the subjects (as in the *vender* and *vivir* charts above).

ordeñar [to milk]	correr [to run (applies to animals or people)]	abrir [open]
cambiar [to change]	beber [to drink]	recibir [receive]
revisar [to check over, look over]	aprender [to learn]	escribir [write]
lavar [to wash]	comprender [to understand]	cubrir [cover]
cuidar [to take care of, watch out for]	deber [ought, should]	decidir [decide]
reparar [to repair]	depender (de) [depend (on)]	reunir [herd]
alimentar [to feed]	creer [believe]*	resistir [resist]
esquilar [to shear]	comer [eat]	añadir [add]
terminar [to finish, end]	absorber [absorb]	consumir [consume]
limpiar [to clean]	toser [cough]	subir [go up]

*For the rest of the table, "to" is omitted from English definitions.

EXERCISE 4-2

What is the Spanish equivalent of the English phrase below?

1. he washes
2. we shear
3. they write
4. you guys should
5. she checks over
6. I receive
7. you (formal) believe
8. Pedro adds
9. the cow coughs
10. Juanita takes care
11. Juan and Ramón open ("and" = *y*)
12. María and I depend
13. I clean
14. you (informal) change
15. Manuel and Lupe milk
16. Carlos and I finish
17. the piglets run
18. the calf consumes
19. you (formal) repair
20. the price goes up ("price" = *el precio*)
21. I understand

CULTURAL NOTE:
FORMAL AND INFORMAL "YOU"

In Spanish, there is both a formal "you" [usted] and an informal "you" [tú]. In the old days, English had different forms too, but "you" (formal) eventually replaced "thou" (informal). How do you know which kind of "you" to use?

Some situations are clearly informal, as, for example, when an adult speaks with children. In that case, the adult would use *tú* with the children, and the children would use *usted* with the adult. Some situations are clearly formal; when you speak with a government official, for example, you should definitely use *usted*. But there are other situations that are not as clear, and as a foreigner to Latino culture, you are not ready to make subtle judgments about those gray areas. Don't panic—you won't go wrong by using the formal *usted* in your normal speech.

To understand why you should use *usted,* keep in mind that Latino culture generally is more formal and courtesy conscious than Anglo culture, especially U.S. culture. (In fact, it's hard to find a more informal culture than that of the United States. Natives of the United States are notorious around the world for being too friendly too soon, which is often interpreted as being pushy.) Because Anglo culture tends to consider "formal" to be a negative term, you might think that using *usted* is cold or distant or snobby. But in Latino culture, "formal" is a positive, attractive term, and the use of formal courtesy is still important at all levels of society. One reason for this heightened awareness of courtesy is that the concept of respect is crucial in Latino society. There are entire books written about this idea and its related concepts of personal dignity and honor, but in practical terms, you should know that it's a smart idea to behave *in obvious ways* to indicate that there is respect and dignity in your dealings with Latinos. Therefore, rushing into using someone's first name or *tú* will probably create a bad impression, while using *usted* will not.

This culture of respect has created a nice spin-off for novice Spanish speakers. No matter how many mistakes you make in your Spanish, trying to speak it is a great gesture of respect. The people you speak with are likely to be patient and helpful with your struggling Spanish. The Anglo coauthor of this book has never witnessed a Latino making fun of an English speaker who was genuinely trying to speak Spanish. Considering the whopping mistakes she made when she was learning Spanish, that's quite a tribute to the ability of Latinos to both recognize good intentions and keep a straight face. There, that took a little pressure off, didn't it?

CHAPTER 5

Weak-Kneed Verbs and "Not" Sentences

Weak-Kneed Verbs

Some Spanish vowels, when they're surrounded by strong, aggressive consonants, fall apart (both in spelling and pronunciation) when the pronounced stress falls on them. Well, we all fall apart under stress, don't we? The *e* in this kind of weak-kneed verb has a habit of breaking down into *ie* or *i*, and the *o* can break down into *ue*. This change doesn't happen to all verbs; it just happens to the weak-kneed ones, and even then the falling apart happens only when the stress falls on the weak link. (If you need to review the stress rules, go back to chapter 1.) In practical terms, weak-kneed verbs fall apart in all forms except the *nosotros* form.

An example of a common weak-kneed verb is *querer* [to want]. The first *e* is the fragile one, which is too bad, because the pronounced stress falls on that weak link in every form except the *nosotros* form. Here's how it looks in its chart:

Querer (ie) [to want]

quiero	queremos
quieres	
quiere	quieren

See how the weak *e* fragments into *ie* when the stress falls on it? Here's another weak-kneed verb, except that in this one, a weak *o* fragments into *ue:*

Volver (ue) [to return]

vuelvo	volvemos
vuelves	
vuelve	vuelven

And here's one that has a weak *e* changing into an *i:*

Pedir (i) [to ask for, to request]

pido	pedimos
pides	
pide	piden

Here are some common weak-kneed verbs, with the weak vowel underlined and the change in parentheses:

to understand	entender (ie)
to begin	comenzar (ie)
to recommend	recomendar (ie)
to lose	perder (ie)
to be able to, can, may	poder (ue)

to cost	c<u>o</u>star (ue)
to sleep	d<u>o</u>rmir (ue)
to count	c<u>o</u>ntar (ue)
to measure	m<u>e</u>dir (i)
to serve	s<u>e</u>rvir (i)
to repeat	rep<u>e</u>tir (i)
to yield, render, produce	r<u>e</u>ndir (i)

EXERCISE 5-1

On a scratch sheet of paper, conjugate the verbs listed above.

EXERCISE 5-2

Change the following phrases to Spanish. (The phrases aren't complete sentences. Later you'll learn how to finish "the veterinarian recommends" to say, "the veterinarian recommends a supplement." For now, just write the verb phrase.) Example: "I understand" = *entiendo.*

1. the chickens sleep
2. we sleep
3. the veterinarian recommends
4. Pablo and Norberto can
5. this sow costs
6. that bull measures
7. you (formal) understand
8. this cow yields
9. Tomás and I count
10. you (informal) lose
11. this restaurant serves ("restaurant" = *el restaurante*)
12. the fair begins ("fair" = *la feria*)
13. the foreman and the inspector repeat
14. the foreman and I repeat

"Not" Sentences

Enough of this positive thinking! Let's be negative! To make a sentence negative, add the word *no* in front of the conjugated verb:

> *Vuelvo tarde.* = I'll be back late.
> *No vuelvo tarde.* – I won't be back late.

> *Estos suplementos cuestan mucho.* = These supplements cost a lot.
> *Estos suplementos no cuestan mucho.* = These supplements don't cost a lot.

> *El nutriólogo recomienda más vitaminas.* = The nutritionist recommends more vitamins.
> *El nutriólogo no recomienda más vitaminas.* = The nutritionist does not recommend more vitamins.

Notice that English often requires the addition of "do" or "does" to its negative sentences. Spanish doesn't require that: its negative sentences are simpler, only requiring that little *no* before the verb.

EXERCISE 5-3

Change the phrases in 5-2 to their negative form. Example: "I don't understand" = *no entiendo.*

1. the chickens don't sleep
2. we don't sleep
3. the veterinarian doesn't recommend
4. Pablo and Norberto can't
5. this sow doesn't cost
6. that bull doesn't measure
7. you (formal) don't understand
8. this cow doesn't yield
9. Tomás and I don't count

10. you (informal) don't lose
11. this restaurant doesn't serve ("restaurant" = *el restaurante*)
12. the fair doesn't begin ("fair" = *la feria*)
13. the foreman and the inspector don't repeat
14. the foreman and I don't repeat

Special Vocabulary: Vehicles ──────────

baler	la empacadora
car	el auto; el carro
chopper	la picadora
combine	la combinada
forklift	el montacargas
harvester	la cosechadora
hay swather	la segadora
loader	el cargador
mixer	la mezcladora
pickup truck	la camioneta; la troca (in the United States)
tractor	el tractor
trailer	el remolque
truck	el camión
wheelbarrow	la carretilla

To run well [*andar bien*]

El auto anda bien. = The car runs well.
Los autos andan bien. = The cars run well.
El auto no anda bien. = The car doesn't run well.
Los autos no andan bien. = The cars don't run well.

To function well [*funcionar bien*]

La mezcladora funciona bien. = The mixer functions well.
Las mezcladoras funcionan bien. = The mixers function well.

La mezcladora no funciona bien. = The mixer doesn't
  function well.
Las mezcladoras no funcionan bien. = The mixers don't
  function well

To run badly [*andar mal*]

El camión anda mal. = The truck runs badly.
Los camiones andan mal. = The trucks run badly.
El camión no anda mal. = The truck doesn't run badly.
Los camiones no andan mal. = The trucks don't run badly.

To function badly [*funcionar mal*]

La computadora funciona mal. = The computer functions
  badly.
Las computadoras funcionan mal. = The computers function
  badly.
La computadora no funciona mal. = The computer doesn't
  function badly.
Las computadoras no funcionan mal. = The computers don't
  function badly.

EXERCISE 5-4

Change the following phrases to Spanish.

1. The combine runs well.
2. The baler doesn't run badly!
3. The tractor doesn't run well.
4. The choppers function well.
5. The harvesters run well.
6. The pickups run well.
7. The forklift doesn't function well.
8. The mixer functions badly.

6

Irregular Verbs

Five Essential Irregular Verbs

It would be too easy if all verbs followed the regular patterns you learned in the previous chapters. So to build your character, there are irregular verbs, that is, verbs that don't follow the neat models laid out in chapters 4 and 5. Among the irregular verbs, there are five essential ones that pop up in every conversation you'll ever have in Spanish. You need to know these verbs very well! You need to memorize and practice them until you can form them without stopping to think.

The first irregular essential verb is *ser*, and it's formed like this:

Ser [to be]

soy [I am]	somos [we are]
eres [you are, informal]	
es [he, she is; you are, formal]	son [they are, ya'll are]

This verb is the equivalent of the English "to be" in the sense of physical appearance, profession, nationality, personality, qualities that don't change, or qualities that someone is born with. This verb can be used in combination with adjectives (such as colors) or nouns (such as professions). Here are some examples of *ser:*

Soy mexicano. = I am Mexican.
Eres Manuel, ¿no? = You're Manuel, aren't you?
El cerdo es negro. = The pig is black.
Somos veterinarios. = We are veterinarians.
Daniel y Pepe son simpáticos. = Daniel and Pepe are nice.
La vida del ranchero es difícil. = A rancher's life is difficult.
Pero es la única vida para mí. = But it's the only life for me.

The second essential irregular verb is *estar,* which also means "to be," but in the sense of conditions that are changeable, such as the weather or health, or conditions that exist because of the results of an action, or a condition that is different from the previous condition. This verb is used with adjectives only:

Estar [to be]

estoy [I am]	estamos [we are]
estás [you are, informal]	
está [he, she is; you are, formal]	están [they are, ya'll are]

Estoy cansado. = I'm tired. (Being tired comes and goes; you aren't born that way. Also, it's the result of an action that made you tired, such as hauling hay all day.)

¿Estás enferma, Elena? = Are you sick, Helen? (Health is changeable; so use *estar* to describe it.)

La oveja está preñada. = The ewe is pregnant. (Pregnancy isn't innate; it comes and goes and is also the result of an action.)

Estamos tristes hoy. = We are sad today. (Emotions such as sadness or happiness are related to *estar* both because they're changeable and because something happened that made you sad or happy. To say that someone has a sad personality or a cheerful personality, use *ser.*)

Los corderos están gordos ahora. = The lambs are fat now. (They used to be underweight and you fed them up to a

nicer weight; for example, you're contrasting their condition
now with their previous condition.)

La gallina está muerta. = The hen is dead. (Being dead is a
change from the previous condition of being alive.)

This next irregular verb is *tener,* meaning "to have" or "to own."
It's used with nouns:

Tener [I have]

tengo [I have]	tenemos [we have]
tienes [you have, informal]	
tiene [he, she has; you have, formal]	tienen [they have, ya'll have]

Tengo doscientas vacas lecheras. = I have 200 milk cows.
Tienes un Ford F-150, ¿no? = You have a Ford F-150, don't
you?
La vaca tiene mastitis. = The cow has mastitis.
Tenemos una venta importante en julio. = We have an important
sale in July.
Los cerdos no tienen suficiente peso. = The hogs don't weigh a
sufficient amount. (Literally, "The hogs don't have sufficient
weight.")

The verb *ir* means "to go." It's followed by *a,* meaning "to." When
a occurs in front of *el,* the two words squish together to make *al.*

Ir [to go]

voy [I go]	vamos [we go]
vas [you go, informal]	
va [he, she goes; you go, formal]	van [they go, ya'll go]

Voy a Chicago para el taller. = I go (or I am going) to
 Chicago for the workshop.
Vas a la farmacia después del almuerzo, ¿no? = You're going
 to the pharmacy after lunch, aren't you?
Manolo va a la granja de los García. = Manolo goes (or is
 going) to the Garcías' farm.
Vamos a la sala de ordeño muy temprano. = We go to the
 milking parlor very early.
Las gallinas van al corral. =The chickens go to the barnyard.

The verb *hay* is the simplest irregular verb of them all. It only has
one form, and that's *hay*. It's everyone's favorite verb, because it's so
simple! It means "there is" or "there are."

Hay [there is, there are]

Hay dos vacas en la carretera. = There are two cows on the
 highway.
Hay gasolina en el camión. = There's gas in the truck.
No hay gasolina en el camión. =There's no gas in the truck.
Hay un problema con el toro nuevo. = There's a problem with
 the new bull.

EXERCISE 6-1

Change the following phrases to Spanish.
Example: "Tina is nice." = *Tina es simpática.*

  1. There is a sale in Omaha.
  2. These hens are sick.
  3. This bull is dangerous. ("dangerous" = *peligroso, peligrosa;*
     a personality problem, not a passing mood)
  4. The herd goes to the creek.
  5. I have a lot of work. ("work" = *el trabajo*)
  6. We are tired!
  7. That ewe is a Merino.
  8. There are salt licks for the goats. ("salt lick" = *la salegar*

or *el saladero;* "for" = *para*)

9. The piglets weigh a sufficient amount (literally, "have sufficient weight").
10. You (formal) go in the pickup.

Now change the sentences to their negative form.
Example: "Tina is not nice." = *Tina no es simpática.*

1. There isn't a sale in Omaha.
2. These hens aren't sick.
3. This bull isn't dangerous.
4. The herd doesn't go to the creek
5. I don't have a lot of work.
6. We are not tired!
7. That ewe is not a Merino.
8. There are no salt licks for the goats.
9. The piglets don't weigh a sufficient amount (literally, "don't have sufficient weight").
10. You (formal) don't go in the pickup. You go in the truck.

Go-Go Irregular Verbs

Some verbs have an irregularity in their *yo* form but are either regular or weak-kneed in their other forms (that is, they are predictable in all the forms except the *yo* one). Often, that irregular *yo* form has the letters *go* at the end (although not always), so we call these verbs the *go-go* verbs as a way to remember them.

hacer (to make, to do) = *hago, haces, hace, hacemos, hacen*
decir (i) (to say, to tell) = *digo, dices, dice, decimos, dicen*
poner (to put, to lay [eggs]) = *pongo, pones, pone, ponemos, ponen*
saber (to know [a fact]) = *sé, sabes, sabe, sabemos, saben*

conocer (to know [a person]) = <u>*conozco*</u>, *conoces, conoce,*
   conocemos, conocen
traer (to bring) = <u>*traigo*</u>, *traes, trae, traemos, traen*
salir (to leave) = <u>*salgo*</u>, *sales, sale, salimos, salen*
venir (ie) (to come) = <u>*vengo*</u>, *vienes, viene, venimos, vienen*
ver (to see) = <u>*veo*</u>, *ves, ve, vemos, ven*

EXERCISE 6-3

Change the following phrases to Spanish.

1. Pablo brings the trailer.
2. I bring the trailer.
3. Jessic and Ray leave late.
4. I leave late.
5. My friends don't know the García family. ("the García family" = *los García*)
6. I don't know the García family.
7. The cows come slowly to the barn. ("slowly" = *despacio*)
8. I come slowly to the barn.
9. The inspectors say that there is no problem. ("that" as a connecting word = *que*)
10. I say that there is no problem.
11. We do our chores. ("chore" = *el quehacer*)
12. I do my chores.
13. You guys put the hay in the pasture.
14. I put the hay in the pasture.
15. The sheep know that they eat soon. ("soon" = *pronto*)
16. I know that I eat soon!

Special Vocabulary: Tools and Equipment

broom, push broom	el cepillo
bucket	el balde, la cubeta
filter	el filtro

fork, pitchfork	la horquilla, el trinchete
funnel	el embudo
halter	el cabestro
hoe	el azadón
hog snare	el asa trompas
hose	la manguera
key	la llave
lasso	el lazo
lock	la cerradura
mop	el estropajo
pump	la bomba
rake	el rastrillo
rope	la soga
scales	la báscula
scraper	el raspador
shovel	la pala
shearing clippers	la esquiladora
siphon	el sifón
towel	la toalla

Some common phrases for usig tools:

Where is the hoe? = *¿Dónde está el azadón?*

It's here. It's over there. = *Está aquí. Está allí.*

I don't know. I haven't seen it. = *No sé. No lo he visto.*

I left it in the pickup. = *Lo dejé en la camioneta.*

Please clean the shovel after using it. = *Por favor, limpie la pala después de usarla.*

Bring the scraper, please. = *Traiga el raspador, por favor.*

Hand me the rope, please. = *Páseme la soga, por favor.*

Clean the trailer with the hose. = *Limpie el remolque con la manguera.*

CULTURAL NOTE: PERSONAL DISTANCE

Sometimes nonverbal acts are as important as verbal ones, although we're often not aware of them. Take, for instance, personal distance. When you're talking with someone, how far away do you stand? Your answer will reflect your native culture. In some cultures, there is considerable distance between speaking partners; in the United States, for example, we like to maintain our "personal space," which can be two to three feet or even more. We don't like to sit in adjoining chairs in theaters, classrooms, or church; when we have the choice, we like to have at least one, and preferably two, empty chairs between us and other individuals or family units. Think of the many phrases in English that emphasize the importance of distance: "too close for comfort," "keep your distance," "don't crowd me."

Are you sensing the potential for culture clash? I hope so, because in Latin culture proper personal space generally falls between twelve and eighteen inches. Many Anglos feel uncomfortable and threatened when someone stands that close! Typically, when groups of Latinos and Anglos are standing around talking, the Anglos are constantly taking a step backward, and the Latinos are constantly taking a step forward. The Anglos are giving off signals of alarm by putting their hands in their pockets, crossing their arms, or turning sideways rather than face to face. The signals increase when a Latino touches the arm of the Anglo during the conversation. These signals communicate to the Latinos the message that the Anglos don't like Latinos. Meanwhile, the Anglos are thinking that Latinos are pushy or grabby. Misunderstandings everywhere!

Next time you're feeling uncomfortable around someone from another culture, try this experiment. Take a step forward or backward, and gauge the resulting comfort or discomfort. If your disquiet is merely a matter of personal distance, you will become aware of it, and you can adjust your thinking accordingly.

CHAPTER 7

Infinitive Phrases and Questions

Infinitive Phrases

Now that you know some verbs, you're ready to learn a very handy little trick to get extra usage out of them: infinitive phrases. Some verbs can be combined with an infinitive to make an idea. For example, I can use *tener* to show that I have a lot of sheep: *tengo muchas ovejas*. But I can also combine *tener* with *que* and another infinitive to make the idea of "have to" (or as we say in conversation, "hafta"): *Tengo que comprar un camión nuevo* [I have to buy a new truck]. Here are some of the most useful infinitive phrases:

- *poder* + infinitive = to be able to
  Podemos hablar español. = We can speak Spanish.

- *acabar de* + infinitive = to have just
  Acabo de pedir unas vitaminas. = I have just ordered some vitamins.

- *ir a* + infinitive = to be going to

  Van a comprar dos vacas. – They are going to buy two cows.

- *querer* + infinitive = to want to

  Quiero terminar temprano. = I want to finish early.

- *deber* + infinitive = to ought to, to should (many people use *deber de* + infinitive)

  Estas vitaminas deben ayudar (or *Estas vitaminas deben de ayudar*). = These vitamins should help.

- *necesitar* + infinitive = to need to

  Estos cerdos necesitan comer más sal. = These pigs need to eat more salt.

- *saber* + infinitive = to know how to

  Paco sabe administrar los primeros auxilios. = Paco knows how to give first aid.

EXERCISE 7-1

Change the following sentences to Spanish. Example: *(vender unos becerros)* I have to sell some calves. = *Tengo que vender unos becerros.*

1. *(comprar un antibiótico)*

I have to buy an antibiotic.
I want to buy an antibiotic.
I can buy an antibiotic.
I am going to buy an antibiotic.
I should buy an antibiotic.
I have just bought an antibiotic.
I need to buy an antibiotic.

2. *(vender unos becerros)*

We should sell some calves.
We have just sold some calves.
We need to sell some calves.
We want to sell some calves.
We can sell some calves.
We are going to sell some calves.
We have to sell some calves.

3. *(entregar el mijo hoy)*

They have to deliver the millet today.
They are going to deliver the millet today.
They need to deliver the millet today.
They can deliver the millet today.
They have just delivered the millet today.
They want to deliver the millet today.
They should deliver the millet today.

4. *(inspeccionar el ganado)*

The veterinarian wants to inspect the cattle.
The veterinarian has just inspected the cattle.
The veterinarian should inspect the cattle.
The veterinarian is going to inspect the cattle.
The veterinarian has to inspect the cattle.
The veterinarian needs to inspect the cattle.
The veterinarian can inspect the cattle.
The veterinarian knows how to inspect the cattle.

5. *(reparar la cerca)*

You (formal) can repair the fence.
You should repair the fence.
You are going to repair the fence.
You want to repair the fence.
You have just repaired the fence.
You have to repair the fence.
You need to repair the fence.
You know how to repair the fence.

6. *(no pagar ese precio)*

I am not going to pay that price.
I do not want to pay that price.
I do not have to pay that price.
I do not need to pay that price.
I should not pay that price.
I cannot pay that price.

Forming Questions

Alas, we don't live only in a world of answers. We humans must ask questions! How do we do that in Spanish? By reversing the order of the subject and the verb from SV to VS:

Jorge habla español. [Jorge speaks Spanish.]
‾‾‾‾‾‾‾‾‾‾‾‾‾
 S   V

¿Habla Jorge español? [Does Jorge speak Spanish?]
‾‾‾‾‾‾‾‾‾‾‾‾
 V   S

Los cerdos prefieren las zanahorias. [The pigs prefer carrots.]
‾‾‾‾‾‾‾‾‾‾‾‾‾‾‾‾‾‾
 S   V

¿Prefieren los cerdos las zanahorias? [Do the pigs prefer carrots?]
‾‾‾‾‾‾‾‾‾‾‾‾‾‾‾‾‾
 V   S

Notice that English needs the helper verb "does" or "do" in order to form a question. Spanish doesn't need that extra word.

EXERCISE 7-2

Change the statement to a question. Example: *Las ovejas necesitan más vitaminas. = ¿Necesitan las ovejas más vitaminas?*

1. *Las gallinas comen mucho sorgo.*
2. *Las cabras rinden mucha leche.*
3. *Usted puede terminar temprano.*
4. *Los becerros son mansos.* (*manso* = "docile," "tame")
5. *Ustedes prefieren las vitaminas orgánicas.*

We often use questioning words to take the place of the unknown information we're seeking. Here are some useful questioning words:

who?	¿quién?
where?	¿dónde?
to where?	¿adónde?
when?	¿cuándo?
how?	¿cómo?
how many?	¿cuánto? (an adjective with male, female, singular, and plural forms)
what?	¿qué?

Here are some question-answer exchanges using the infinitive phrases you've just learned.

¿Qué idiomas pueden ustedes hablar? = What languages can you guys speak?

Podemos hablar español. = We can speak Spanish.

¿Cuántas vacas van a comprar? = How many cows are they going to buy?

Van a comprar dos vacas. = They are going to buy two cows.

¿Cuándo quieres terminar hoy? = When do you want to finish today?

Quiero terminar temprano. = I want to finish early.

¿Cómo progresan los cerdos nuevos? = How are the new pigs progressing?

Los cerdos necesitan comer más sal. = The pigs need to eat more salt.

¿Quién tiene que trabajar el domingo? = Who has to work on Sunday?

Jorge tiene que trabajar el domingo. = Jorge has to work Sunday.

¿Dónde debemos poner las salegares? = Where should we put the salt licks?

Ustedes deben poner las salegares en el pastizal del norte. = You guys should put the salt licks in the north pasture.

EXERCISE 7-3

Change the following questions to Spanish. Example: "Who milks tomorrow?" = *¿Quién ordeña mañana?*

1. When does the veterinarian arrive? ("to arrive" = *llegar*)
2. Where should I put the new hogs?
3. How much milk does this cow yield?
4. How do the cattle respond to the cottonseed cakes? (to "respond" = *responder*)
5. How many bales do you (formal) need?

Although you no doubt know the answers to all such questions, other people might not know them. Here are some handy phrases for those puzzled people:

No sé. = I don't know.
No estoy seguro. = I'm not sure (masculine).
No estoy segura. = I'm not sure (feminine).
¿Quién sabe? = Who knows?
No tengo idea. = I have no idea.
Creo que… = I think that…

EXERCISE 7-4

Answer the questions in exercise 7-3, using the phrases above for not knowing. Example: *¿Quién ordeña mañana?* = *Creo que Manuel va a ordeñar mañana.*

1. Who knows? His pickup is broken down. ("to be broken down" = *estar descompuesto*)
2. I don't know. Maybe in the north pasture? ("maybe" = *quizás*)
3. I'm not sure. Camareno has the logbook. ("logbook" = *la bitácora*)
4. I think that they prefer alfalfa.
5. I have no idea. Maybe three or four.

Special Vocabulary: Machinery ─────────────

applicator	el aplicador
dipping vat	el baño de inmersión
escape valve; relief valve	la válvula de escape, la válvula de seguridad
faucet; wrench	la llave
feeder	el comedero
feed mill	el molino de alimento
heater	el calentador
loader; forklift	el montacargas
machinery	la maquinaria
manure spreader	la esparcidora de estiércol
milking machine	la ordeñadora
nozzle	la boquilla
pasteurizer	la pasterizadora
pipe	el tubo, la caña
pump	la bomba
separator	la descremadora
sprayer	el rociador
tank	el tanque
valve	la válvula

8

Giving: The Verb *Dar*

The verb "to give" is *dar,* and it's conjugated like the verb *ir.*

Dar [to give]

yo doy	nosotros damos
tú das	
él, ella, usted da	ellas, ellos, ustedes dan

Sentences with *Dar*

Notice that you can't make a complete sentence out of just *doy* [I give]. There are parts missing: *What* do you give? And to *whom* do you give it? The concept of giving includes three elements that relate to each other: the giver, the object being given, and the receiver. Let's say that I want to give Juan the keys to the truck. Who is the giver? I am. What is being given? The keys. Who receives the keys? Juan.

Notice that the grammar-conscious writers of the paragraph above wrote, "To *whom* do you give it?" but English speakers don't really say "whom" out loud these days in ordinary speech. That's too bad, in a way, because "whom" clearly shows that it's a receiver, not a doer. It's important to be clear about who's doing what to whom; we observers like to know the difference between "John gives Mary a kiss" and "Mary gives John a kiss." English labels its receiver by positioning it after the verb, and the giver is labeled by positioning it before the verb.

Spanish has a different system of labeling givers, objects, and receivers. You already know that the giver (the actor or the subject) and the verb work together in the opening parts of the sentence:

yo doy or simply *doy*

Now add the object being given after the verb. In the case of "I give Juan the keys," the object is "keys," in Spanish, *las llaves:*

Doy <u>las llaves</u>.

Now we need to add the second person, Juan, who is the receiver, and we want to make sure that we don't get him mixed up with the giver. So, let's add the word *le* [to him] in front of the verb and put the labeler *a* in front of Juan's name:

<u>*Le*</u> *doy las llaves <u>a</u> Juan.*

If you've already mentioned the name "Juan," so that the person you're talking to knows whom you're talking about, you can just say, "I give the keys to him":

<u>*Le*</u> *doy las llaves.*

And that's a good Spanish sentence. I know, I know, it's not like English. I know, I know, you think that English is simpler. Well, Spanish speakers think that Spanish is simpler—and clearer!

EXERCISE 8-1

Change the following sentences to Spanish, using the verb *dar.* Example: *Manuel* (giver), *la alfalfa* ("alfalfa," the object), *la vaca* (receiver) = *Manuel le da la alfalfa a la vaca.*

1. *Carlos* (giver), *el maíz* ("corn," object), *el cerdo* (receiver)
2. *María* (giver), *las vitaminas* ("vitamins," object),
   la gallina (receiver)
3. *Ramón* (giver), *los suplementos* ("supplements," object),
   la oveja (receiver)
4. *Pablo y yo* (givers), *el calcio* ("calcium," object),
   a vaca (receiver)
5. *Francisco y Martín* (givers), *el heno* ("hay," object),
   el toro (receiver)

Check your answers in the answer key at the back of this book. Did you follow the pattern pretty well? Now try this follow-up exercise:

EXERCISE 8-2

Change the following sentences to Spanish. Example: "Manuel gives it *(la vaca)* alfalfa" = *Manuel le da la alfalfa.*

1. Carlos gives it *(el cerdo)* the corn.
2. María gives it *(la gallina)* the vitamins.
3. Ramón gives it *(la oveja)* the supplements.
4. Pablo and I give it *(la vaca)* the calcium.
5. Francisco and Martín give it *(el toro)* the hay.

What if the receiver is plural? Then change *le* to *les.*

EXERCISE 8-3

Change the following sentences to Spanish. Example: "Manuel gives them *(las vacas)* alfalfa" = *Manuel les da la alfalfa.*

1. Carlos gives them *(los cerdos)* the corn.
2. María gives them *(las gallinas)* the vitamins.
3. Ramón gives them *(las ovejas)* the supplements.
4. Pablo and I give them *(las vacas)* the calcium.
5. Francisco and Martín give them *(los toros)* the hay.

Now let's play with the sentence "Jaime gives _____
the report." The word for "report" in Spanish is *el informe,* and it's our
object. Jaime is the giver. You already know the receiver *le.* Now let's
add these receivers:

to me	me
to you (informal)	te
to us	nos
to them	les
to ya'll, to you guys	les

These receivers fit into the same slot as *le* in exercise 8-2 and *les* in
exercise 8-3.

EXERCISE 8-4

Change the following sentences to Spanish. Example: "Jaime gives
him the report." = *Jaime le da el informe.*

1. Jaime gives us the report.
2. Jaime gives me the report.
3. Jaime gives them the report.
4. Jaime gives you (informal) the report.
5. Jaime gives you guys the report.
6. Jaime gives Hernán and me the report.
7. Jaime gives Karen the report.
8. Jaime gives Hernán and Karen the report.

Are you starting to feel the pattern? Let's practice some more, adding
some more verbs that, like *dar,* require an object and a receiver. These
verbs are all regular.

EXERCISE 8-5

Form a sentence using the following elements. Example:

doer	verb	object	receiver	complete sentence
Jaime	dar	el informe	María	Jaime le da el informe a María.

doer	verb	object	receiver or the person who benefits	complete sentence
yo	comprar [to buy]	rosas [roses]	Mamá	1.
Carmen	enviar [to send]	el cheque [the check]	el vendedor [the buyer]	2.
el señor Jones	vender [to sell]	la avena	yo	3.
Nina	mostrar [to show] weak-kneed verb, *o* to *ue*	el rancho	los socios del club FFA [members of the FFA club]	4.
ustedes	dar [to give]	sus raciones	las gallinas	5.
Miguel y yo	cortar [to cut, clip]	las uñas [the nails]	los cerditos	6.
el señor Hernández	esquilar [to shear]	la lana [the wool]	nosotros	7.
usted	prestar [to loan]	su navaja [your pocketknife]	Mario	8.
el inspector	escribir [to write]	su informe	usted	9.
nosotros	entregar [to turn in, hand over]	las cuentas [the accounts]	la contadora [the (female) accountant]	10.

Special Vocabulary: Feed
(part 1—see chapter 9 for part 2)

alfalfa	la alfalfa
apple	la manzana
barley	la cebada
carrot	la zanahoria
cereal	el cereal
clover	el trébol
corn	el maíz
fodder	el forraje; el pienso
food, feeding, nourishment	la alimentación
grain	el grano
grass	el pasto, la hierba
grazing	el pastoreo
hay	el heno
mash	el puré
millet	el mijo, el millo
oats	la avena
prickly pear cactus	el nopal (in Mexico), la tuna
ration	la ración
ryegrass	el ballico, or *"ryegrass"*
sedum	la hierba callera
silage	el ensilaje
sorghum	el sorgo
vetch	la veza

CHAPTER 9

Shorthand for Objects

Objects are things or people in the sentence that are neither the doer (the subject) nor the receiver. You saw some objects in the previous chapter when you learned how to construct giving-type sentences: "Juan gives <u>inoculations</u> to the ewes." Objects can occur in lots of sentences, not just giving-type ones. For example, there are objects in these sentences:

> Do you have the <u>keys</u>? ("Keys" is neither a doer nor a
>   receiver; the doer is "you," and there is no receiver.)
> I know <u>her.</u>
> We stacked <u>the bales</u> over there.
> They buy <u>cattle</u> at the auction in Fort Worth.
> He inspected the <u>feeder pigs</u>.
> I phone <u>Mom</u> every Sunday.

When you learned verb conjugations by themselves ("I speak," "they buy") without objects, they probably sounded funny. The phrases were too short; they seemed incomplete. We don't use many verbs alone without some sort of elaboration. One of the most common ways to complete the verb phrase is to add an object, as the examples above indicate.

EXERCISE 9-1

Underline the object in each of the following sentences. Example: "Jessie repairs the fence." = "Jessie repairs <u>the fence</u>."

    1. Manuel milks the cow.
    2. Pablo and Ramón shear the sheep.
    3. We unload the bales.
    4. They want to buy a new trailer.
    5. Do you have the shovel?
    6. We clean the stalls every day.
    7. You weigh the lambs often.
    8. You should read the instructions.
    9. The cows break the fence.
  10. I sterilize the equipment.

EXERCISE 9-2

Now change the sentences above to Spanish. Example: "Jessie repairs the fence" = *Jessie repara la cerca.*

    1. Manuel milks the cow.
    2. Pablo and Ramón shear the sheep.
    3. We unload the bales.
    4. They want to buy a new trailer.
    5. Do you have the shovel?
    6. We clean the stalls every day.
    7. You (formal) weigh the lambs often.
    8. You (formal) should read the instructions.
    9. The cows break the fence.
  10. I sterilize the equipment.

We use objects so much that we often use brief forms of them; that is, we don't always repeat the whole object every time we say it. For example, what's wrong with this conversation?

    "Dad, do you have the newspaper?"

"No, I don't have the newspaper. Perhaps your mother has
    the newspaper."
"I already asked her about the newspaper. She says you have
    the newspaper."

Right, too many "newspapers." We don't talk like this, either in
English or Spanish. Instead, once we've identified the object, we use
a brief form, a shorthand form, for it afterward. Here is a more normal version of the conversation, this time using shorthand forms:

"Dad, do you have the newspaper?"
"No, I don't have it. Perhaps your mother has it."
"I already asked her. She says you have it."

In this case, "it" is the shorthand way of saying "newspaper." Once
the word "newspaper" is used, "it" can take its place subsequently, as
long as you are still speaking to the same person. But if you leave Dad
to go talk to Mom, you'll have to mention "newspaper" once, so that
she'll know what you're talking about.

Here are the shorthand forms of objects:

• Talking about a masculine thing or person, use *lo*.
    The plural form is *los*.
• Talking about a feminine thing or person, use *la*.
    The plural form is *las*.
• When "I" becomes an object, use *me* (don't pronounce it
    like the English "me!").
• When "we" becomes an object, use *nos*.
• When the informal "you" becomes an object, use *te*.

The shorthand object is positioned immediately before the conjugated
verb or, if there's an infinitive in the sentence, stuck onto the end of
the infinitive. Examples:

I have the shovel. = *Tengo la pala.*
I have it. = *La tengo.*
I don't have it. = *No la tengo.*
I want to buy the shovel. = *Quiero comprar la pala.*
I want to buy it. = *Quiero comprarla.*

I don't want to buy it. = *No quiero comprarla.*

I have the shovels. = *Tengo las palas.*
I have them. = *Las tengo.*
I don't have them. = *No las tengo.*
I want to buy them. = *Quiero comprarlas.*
I don't want to buy them. = *No quiero comprarlas.*

Catalina knows us. = *Catalina nos conoce.*
Catalina knows me. = *Catalina me conoce.*
Catalina knows you (informal). = *Catalina te conoce.*

EXERCISE 9-3

Rewrite the sentences you wrote in exercise 9-2, this time using the shorthand form of the object. Example: *Jessie repara la cerca.* = *Jessie la repara.*

   1.
   2.
   3.
   4.
   5.
   6.
   7.
   8.
   9.
   10.

EXERCISE 9-4

Answer the question, using the appropriate shorthand form in your answer. Example: *¿Tiene usted las llaves?* [Do you have the keys?] = *Sí, las tengo.* [Yes, I have them.]

1. ¿Vende usted el heno?
2. ¿Ve usted la cerda Duroc?
3. ¿Quieren ustedes organizar la competición?
4. ¿Conoce usted a los hermanos Santana? (*hermano* = "brother")
5. ¿Puede usted tatuar las ovejas? (*tatuar* = "to tattoo")
6. ¿Todavía tenemos los recibos de AgriChem? (*todavía* = "still"; *el recibo* = "the receipt")
7. ¿Dónde debemos descargar el millo? (*descargar* = "to unload")
8. ¿Busca usted las botellas? (*buscar* = "to search for"; *la botella* = "bottle")
9. ¿Necesitamos al veterinario?
10. ¿Habla usted español?

EXERCISE 9-5

Now change your answers to 9-4 to a negative response. Example: *¿Tiene usted las llaves?* = *No, no las tengo.* [No, I don't have them.]

1. ¿Vende usted el heno?
2. ¿Ve usted la cerda Duroc?
3. ¿Quieren ustedes organizar la competición?
4. ¿Conoce usted a los hermanos Santana?
5. ¿Puede usted tatuar las ovejas?
6. ¿Todavía tenemos los recibos de AgriChem? (Include yourself in the answer's subject.)
7. ¿Dónde debemos descargar el millo? (Don't include yourself in the answer's subject.)
8. ¿Busca usted las botellas?
9. ¿Necesitamos al veterinario? (Include yourself in the answer's subject.)
10. ¿Habla usted español?

Special Vocabulary: Feed (part 2) _____

amino acid	el aminoácido
bonemeal	la harina de huesos
brewer's yeast	la levadura de cerveza
calcium	el calcio
cod liver oil	el aceite de hígado de bacalao
concentrate	el concentrado
cottonseed cake	la torta de algodón
grits	la sémola
iodine	el yodo
iron	el hierro
magnesium	el magnesio
milk	la leche
molasses	la melaza
oil cake	la torta oleaginosa
pellets	los pelets
salt	la sal
salt lick	la salegar *or* el saladero
supplements	los suplementos
vitamins	las vitaminas

CHAPTER 10

Commands

A normal part of conversation consists of giving polite commands, such as "Pick me up at eight," "Pass me the salt," and "Hand me that wrench." This requesting speech is formed by using switched endings. You have previously learned that -*ar* verbs use endings that incorporate the letter *a*, and that -*er* and -*ir* verbs incorporate the letter *e*. Well, for commands, let's switch that, and use *e* for -*ar* verbs and *a* for -*er* and -*ir* verbs. Here's how to form commands:

Regular Commands

- Take the *yo* form of the verb *hablar* [to speak], which is *hablo*. Break off the *o*. Add the switched ending for polite commands, and you get *hable*, as in *Hable más despacio, por favor* [Speak more slowly, please].

To give a command to more than one person, use the ending *en:* *hablen*.

- For the verb *añadir* [to add], start with the *yo* form of *añado*, break off the *o*, add the switched ending *a*, and you get the command *añada*, as in *Añada este suplemento a su dieta* [Add this supplement to its diet]. The plural: *añadan*.

- For the verb *correr* [to run], follow the procedure above to produce the command *corra,* as in *Corra a la casa* [Run to the house!], and *corran,* as in *Corran ustedes a la casa* [Y'all run to the house!].
- If you want a negative command, just put *no* in front: *no hable, no hablen, no añada, no añadan, no corra, no corran.*

Notice that if the *yo* form is irregular (see chapter 6), the command probably is too (exceptions below). For example, to make the command form of the verb *tener,* start with *tengo,* which produces the form *tenga,* as in *Tenga cuidado con los pesticidas* [Be careful—literally—"Have a care with the pesticides"]. The weak-kneed verbs (see chapter 5) will have their fragmented sound in the command, because it occurs in the *yo* form: *volver* becomes *vuelvo* and then *vuelva,* as in *Vuelvan ustedes mañana* [Y'all come back tomorrow].

Irregular Commands _____

Just to keep things lively, there are some irregular commands you'll just have to memorize. Here are four common ones.

ser = sea, sean: Sea profesional con sus clientes.
    [Be professional with your clients.]
estar = esté, estén: Esté tranquilo; la cerda va a sobrevivir.
    [Be calm; the sow will live.]
ir = vaya, vayan: Vaya a la farmacia Cruz Roja.
    [Go to the Red Cross pharmacy.]
dar = dé, den: No le dé más manzanas.
    [Don't give it—e.g., the pig—more apples.]

EXERCISE 10-1

Make commands, positive and negative, of the following verbs. Example: *vivir = viva, no viva, vivan, no vivan.*

1. limpiar [to clean]

2. traer [to bring; a go-go verb]
3. cubrir [to cover]
4. reparar [to repair]
5. poner [to put; a go-go verb]
6. abrir [to open]
7. esterilizar [to sterilize]
8. trabajar [to work]
9. subir [to go up]
10. reunir [to herd]
11. hacer [to do, to make; a go-go verb]
12. cerrar (ie) [to close]
13. medir (i) [to measure]
14. cortar [to cut, to clip]
15. preparar [to prepare]

EXERCISE 10-2

Change these commands to Spanish. Example: "Drink more water" = *Beba más agua.*

1. Clean the stall.
2. Repair the milking machine.
3. Bring the rope.
4. Add more barley.
5. Go to the stable.
6. Inspect the hooves.
7. Come back tomorrow.
8. Count the lambs.
9. Open the gate.
10. Close the gate.

EXERCISE 10-3

Now change the commands to their negative form. Example: "Don't drink more water." = *No beba más agua.*

1. Don't clean the stall.

2. Don't repair the milking machine.
3. Don't bring the rope.
4. Don't add more barley.
5. Don't go to the stable.
6. Don't inspect the hooves.
7. Don't come back tomorrow.
8. Don't count the lambs.
9. Don't open the gate.
10. Don't close the gate.

CHAPTER 11

More about Commands

Commands with Objects

Positive commands attract words such as the giving label or the object shorthand (chapter 9), fastening them on at the end of the command. But negative commands repel those words, pushing them back to their normal position in front. Take a look at these examples:

Déme la esquiladora (dé + me). = Give me the clippers.
No me dé la esquiladora. = Don't give me the clippers.

Dígame las noticias (diga + me). = Tell me the news.
No me diga las noticias. = Don't tell me the news.

Póngalo allí (ponga + lo). = Put it there.
No lo ponga allí. = Don't put it there.

EXERCISE 11-1

Change the following to commands, both positive and negative. Example: *darle una zanahoria a la cabra* [give a carrot to the goat] = *déle una zanahoria a la cabra, no le dé una zanahoria a la cabra.*

1. esquilar la lana
2. tatuarle la oreja al carnero
3. cerrar la puerta
4. terminar los quehaceres
5. prestarle la camioneta a Keith
6. lavar el suelo
7. revisar las llantas
8. repartirles el alambre a los trabajadores
9. darles el antibiótico a los becerros
10. romper la botella

Commands, even polite ones, tend to be short; they don't waste words. Of course, the first time we mention something, we have to say the whole thing: "Don't give the carrot to the goat." But once we establish what we're talking about, we're briefer: "Son, I told you, don't give it to him." That very short phrase, "it to him," is a combination of the receiving labeler and the shorthand object. How do we say that in Spanish? Put the receiver first, followed by the object:

Basic sentence: *El inspector me envía el informe mañana.* = The inspector will send me the report tomorrow.

Command with receiver attached to the command: *Inspector, envíeme el informe mañana.* = Inspector, send me the report tomorrow.

Command with receiver and object attached: *Inspector, envíemelo mañana.* = Inspector, send it to me tomorrow.

Negative command, with no attachments: *Inspector, no me lo envíe mañana.* = Inspector, don't send it to me tomorrow.

Here are the possible combinations of receivers and objects:

me lo, me los, me la, me las
te lo, te los, te la, te las
nos lo, nos los, nos la, nos las

Something funny happens, though, when the combination has two words starting with *l* next to each other. That's a tricky combination in Spanish, so the first word changes to *se* rather than *le*.

No: *le lo!* Yes: *se lo, se los, se la, se las.*

EXERCISE 11-2

Change the following commands to Spanish according to this pattern: "Tell me the problem." = *Dígame el problema. No me diga el problema. Dígamelo. No me lo diga.*

1. Lend her the rake.
   Don't lend her the rake.
   Lend it to her.
   Don't lend it to her.
2. Give me the hose.
   Don't give me the hose.
   Give it to me.
   Don't give it to me.
3. Give him the keys.
   Don't give him the keys.
   Give them to him.
   Don't give them to him.
4. Bring us the wheelbarrow.
   Don't bring us the wheelbarrow.
   Bring it to us.
   Don't bring it to us.
5. Change the bed for the ewes.
   Don't change the bed for the ewes.
   Change it for them.
   Don't change it for them.
   (In this case, express "for the ewes" with the receiver;
      you don't have to include a word for "for.")

6. Show him the logbook.
   Don't show him the logbook.
   Show it to him.
   Don't show it to him.
7. Sell them the trailer.
   Don't sell them the trailer.
   Sell it to them.
   Don't sell it to them.
8. Send her the reports.
   Don't send her the reports.
   Send them to her.
   Don't send them to her.
9. Tell us (you plural) the joke.
   Don't tell us the joke.
   Tell it to us.
   Don't tell it to us.
10. Lend me a dollar.
    Don't lend me a dollar.
    Lend it to me.
    Don't lend it to me.

Double-Commands

Here's a frequently used type of command: Tell Mike to call the vet. It's really two commands: "Tell Mike" + "call the vet." Here's how this double-command looks in Spanish:

Dígale a Mike que llame al veterinario.

Notice that the two commands are linked with the word *que*. If you already know that you're talking about Mike, you don't have to repeat his name:

Dígale que llame al veterinario. = Tell him to call the vet.

The second command can be negative:

> *Dígale que no llame al veterinario.* = Tell him not to call the vet.

The command can be plural too:

> *Dígales a Hernán y Matías que reparen la cerca.* = Tell Hernán and Matías to mend the fence.
> *Dígales que reparen la cerca.* = Tell them to mend the fence.

EXERCISE 11-3

Change the following double-commands to Spanish:

1. Tell Jack to close the door.
2. Tell Jack not to close the door.
3. Tell him to wash the truck.
4. Tell him not to wash the truck.
5. Tell Lupe to buy more ointment.
6. Tell Lupe not to buy more ointment.
7. Tell her to bring me a wrench.
8. Tell her not to bring me a wrench.
9. Tell Miguel and Arón to help me.
10. Tell them to help me.

Suggestions: Alternatives to Commands _____

As useful as commands are, sometimes a suggestion would be better. To make a suggestion, you still use the command form, but you introduce it with a phrase that suggests rather than tells. In this case, the receiver and the shorthand words don't stick to the verb; they go in front of it, as in a noncommand sentence.

> Command: *Déle más vitaminas* = Give it more vitamins.
> Suggestion: *Sugiero que usted le dé más vitaminas.* =
> I suggest that you give it more vitamins.

Command: *No le dé más vitaminas.* = Don't give it more
vitamins.
Suggestion: *Sugiero que no le dé más vitaminas.* = I suggest
that you not give it more vitamins.

Both the commands and the suggestions are proper grammatically,
and they are both proper in terms of etiquette as well, especially when
you say the command in a normal tone of voice and add *por favor*
from time to time. But there are situations when a suggestion is more
appropriate than a command, and you should learn both expressions
so that you can employ them with good judgment. Here are some
more suggestion-type phrases:

> *Es importante que...* = It's important that...
> *Es necesario que...* = It's necessary that...
> *Prefiero que...* = I prefer that...

EXERCISE 11-4

Give the command and the suggestion for each of these phrases.
Example: *Terminar el tatuaje hoy.* = *Termine el tatuaje hoy. Es importante
que termine el tatuaje hoy.*

1. limpiar el tanque
2. añadir agua al bebedero
3. comprar gasolina para la camioneta
4. tener cuidado con los corderos recién nacidos
5. cuidar de la vaca enferma
6. trabajar más rápido
7. ir a la clínica
8. escribir las notas en la bitácora
9. lavarlo con el desinfectante
10. separar las gallinas menos productivas (*menos* = "less")
11. examinar las patas
12. ponerlos en el corral
13. moverlos a otro pastizal
14. cortar las alas
15. acariciarlos

CULTURAL NOTE: POLITE PHRASES

Most of our conversation is supposed to convey information of some sort. But there's another part of ordinary speech that isn't about information at all; it's about sweetening the interaction between humans with courtesy. Don't underestimate the importance of these courteous phrases! They can make the difference between a pleasant working environment and a tense one.

Please = *por favor.* (*Limpie el remolque, por favor.* = "Clean the trailer, please.")

Thank you. = *Gracias.*

Thanks a lot. – *Muchas gracias*

I'm sorry. = *Lo siento* (said after stepping on someone's toe, for example).

Pardon me. = *Perdóneme* (said after bumping into someone, for example).

It's nothing. = *De nada.* Or, *No hay de qué.*

Muy amable. = How kind. (said in reply to a compliment)

What? = *¿Cómo?* Or, *¿Mande?* (in Mexico)
(Note that *¿qué?* by itself is a little rude.)

Repeat, please. = *Repita, por favor.*

Look = *Mire.*

Do it like this. = *Así se hace.* (literally, "Thus it is done," a phrase that doesn't put the person on the spot the way a direct phrase like *Hágalo así* might)

Well done. = *Bien hecho.*

You work well. = *Usted trabaja bien.*

You worked hard today. = *Usted trabajó duro hoy.*

How are you? = *¿Cómo está usted?*

How are you today? = *¿Cómo está hoy?*

How are you today? = *¿Cómo amaneció?* (literally, "How did you dawn?")

Fine, thanks. = *Bien, gracias.*

And you? = *¿Y usted?*

See you tomorrow. = *Hasta mañana.*

Have a nice weekend. = *Que pase bien el fin de semana.*

Have a nice vacation. = *Que pase bien las vacaciones.*

Can you help me, please? = *¿Me puede ayudar, por favor?*

Would you be so kind to… = *¿Sería tan amable de…?*
(This phrase may sound overly polite to English speakers, but it's frequently used in Spanish.)

Would you be so kind as to open the door? = *¿Sería tan amable de abrir la puerta?*

CHAPTER 12

Before-Now Verbs

Regular Before-Now Verbs ─────────────

It's the end of the day, and you're mentally listing the things that you have accomplished up to this point: I have mended the stall, I have doctored the ewe's ear, I have unloaded the feed that was delivered, and on and on. Notice that you "have done" these things. When we use that phrase, we're talking about what happened before now or prior to this moment when we're talking. This is called the "present perfect" in grammar lingo, not because these verbs are better than other verbs, but because in Latin "perfect" means "already done." These are the "already done" or "done before now" or "prior to now" verbs. Good news: the Spanish "before-now" verbs are just like the English ones! If you can use the English ones, you can use the Spanish ones too. So breathe a sigh of relief, and then learn these very useful and very easy verbs.

As in English, the before-now verbs consist of two parts. The "has" or "have" part is expressed by the verb *haber,* which is conjugated like this:

Haber [has, have]

yo he	nosotros hemos
tú has	
él, ella, usted ha	ellos, ellas, ustedes han

Don't pronounce the *h!* And don't prolong the pronunciation of the vowel; say it crisply and shortly.

The second part is called the participle (more grammar lingo). To form it, drop off the infinitive ending, and add *ado* for *-ar* verbs, and *ido* for *-er* and *-ir* verbs.

> *hablar* = *he hablado, has hablado, ha hablado, hemos hablado, han hablado*
> I have spoken, you have spoken, she/he/you has/have spoken, we have spoken, they/y'all have spoken

> *comer* = *he comido, has comido, ha comido, hemos comido, han comido*
> I have eaten, you have eaten, she/he/you has/have eaten, we have eaten, they/y'all have eaten

> *vivir* = *he vivido, has vivido, ha vivido, hemos vivido, han vivido*
> I have lived, you have lived, she/he/you has/have lived, we have lived, they/y'all have lived

The before-now verbs are often accompanied by extra little bits of information such as *ya* [already, still], *todavía* [still], *antes* [before], *siempre* [always], *nunca* [never], *hasta ahora* [until now], or *finalmente* [finally]. As always, to make the sentence negative, just insert *no* into the slot before the conjugated verb: *Ya no he terminado* [I still haven't finished].

EXERCISE 12-1

Conjugate the following verbs in the before-now way.

lavar	comer	venir
reparar	traer	repartir
terminar	leer	recibir
limpiar	recoger	decidir
preparar	mover	reunir

Irregular Participles ─────────────────────

Are there irregular before-now verbs? Of course! These common participles are irregular:

> *hacer = hecho: he hecho, has hecho, ha hecho, hemos hecho, han hecho*
> *decir = dicho*
> *abrir = abierto*
> *cubrir = cubierto*
> *escribir = escrito*
> *morir = muerto*
> *romper = roto*
> *ver = visto*
> *volver = vuelto*
> *poner = puesto*

EXERCISE 12-2

Conjugate the irregular verbs above in the before-now way.

EXERCISE 12-3

Fill in the blank with the proper form of the before-now verb, according to the context. Example: *Mi familia y yo <u>hemos vivido</u> (vivir) en Nebraska muchos años.*

1. Este carnero nunca _____ (ser) peligroso.
2. Hasta ahora, esta máquina siempre _____ (funcionar) bien.
3. Las cerdas _____ (progresar) mucho con la dieta nueva.
4. El rebaño _____ (consumir) más alimentación que antes. (*que antes* = "than before")
5. ¿ _____ (pesar) usted los cabritos?
6. Yo no _____ (hacer) nada hoy. (*nada* = "nothing")
7. Jorge y Fernando, ¿ _____ (poner) ustedes el ganado en el remolque?
8. Yo todavía no _____ (registrar) el progreso de los novillos.
9. Nosotros _____ (comprar) unas cabras nuevas. El veterinario no las _____ (examinar) todavía, pero _____ (*prometer* = "to promise") venir mañana.

EXERCISE 12-4

Change the following sentences to Spanish. Example: *(vivir)* "We have lived here three years." = *Hemos vivido aquí tres años.*

1. *(vender)* Antonio has sold six heifers.
2. *(dormir)* I think that they have slept late!
3. *(separar)* Eduardo has separated the calves for branding.
4. *(limpiar)* Have you cleaned the machinery already?
5. *(terminar; comenzar)* I have not finished the report yet. I haven't begun it!
6. *(salir)* Luisa has left already.

7. *(poder)* We have not been able to repair the separator.
8. *(morir)* The old ewe has died.
9. *(recomendar; comprar)* The vet has recommended more calcium. Have you bought it yet?
10. *(ver)* Have you seen my keys? ("key" = *la llave*)
11. *(llegar)* Finally, the truck with the corn has arrived. ("with" = *con*)
12. *(volver)* Has José returned yet?
13. *(leer, entender)* I have read the instructions, but I have not understood them. ("instructions" = *las instrucciones*; "but" = *pero*)
14. *(subir)* The price has always gone up.
15. *(rendir, esperar)* This cow has not yielded as much milk as I had hoped. ("as much" = *tanto, tanta*; "as" = *como*)

CULTURAL NOTE: THE FAMILY

Family in Latino culture has an importance that Anglos find hard to grasp. For one thing, the word itself means different things in the two cultures. When English speakers say the word "family," they tend to have a mental picture of parents and children (the "nuclear family," as the sociologists say). When Spanish speakers say, "family," they see parents, children, grandparents, aunts and uncles, cousins, godparents, and godchildren; researchers call it the "extended family network." Latino families tend to live in the same neighborhoods, and it's not unusual for one or more relatives to live in the house with the nuclear family. The family members often gather for meals, parties, and outings, such as going to the park on Sunday afternoons. Big decisions—such as whether to purchase land, send kids to college, or take a job—are typically discussed by the entire family. The oldest female's opinion is carefully taken into consideration. Younger brothers will often defer to the oldest brother. If moving to another place is desirable, it is common to send a couple of relatives to the area first, and if it works out, other family members (sometimes lots of family members) will follow. When a Latino goes home to visit family, a little present must be taken to each one of the members of the network.

We could go on, but you probably have the picture by now: families in Latino culture are very, very important. So it should not surprise you that inquiring after the family is a polite thing to do. Inevitably, it is a topic that will come out in conversation. If you show courteous interest in someone's family, they will happily overlook any grammatical errors you make in Spanish.

Let's say that you are meeting your coworkers at the beginning of the workday. As people arrive, it's the custom to comment on the weather (see chapter 15) and inquire about the family: How's the new baby? How did your child do in the baseball game last night? Is your mother feeling better? These questions don't pry into intimate business, they just acknowledge the family and show respect. Here are a few small-talk inquiries about family:

How is your ...?	¿Cómo está su...?
aunt	
baby	el bebé (male);
	la bebita (female)
brother	hermano
cousin (female)	prima
cousin (male)	primo
daughter	hija
family	familia
father	padre
granddaughter	nieta
grandson	nieto
husband	marido
mother	mamá
nephew	sobrino

niece	sobrina
sister	hermana
son	hijo
uncle	tío
wife	esposa

Another way of saying the same thing: *¿Cómo se encuentra su familia?* = literally, "How do you find your family?" As in "Do you find that they are doing well?"

¿Está mejor su <u>mamá</u>? = Is your <u>mother</u> better?
¿Le gusta a su <u>hija</u> la escuela? = Does your <u>daughter</u> like school?
Vi a su <u>hijo</u> ayer. ¡Es casi un hombre ya! = I saw your <u>son</u> yesterday. He's almost a man already!
Su <u>hijo/hija</u> jugó bien en el partido anoche. = Your <u>son/daughter</u> played well in the game last night.

How will you know what the answer is? By the expression on the person's face. If the mother is better, there will be a hopeful look on the face. If the child doesn't like school, the look will be rueful. The comment about the son will probably produce a proud look, even if the son is driving the parents crazy. The Spanish speaker will respond to your inquiries with general answers, suitable for small talk, so don't worry about complicated grammar. The grammar of facial expressions and tones of voice will take over in this situation.

What if the Spanish speaker asks about your family? Give the same general answers, accompanied by smiles, laughs, rolling the eyes, shrugs, shaking the head.

Bien, gracias. = Fine, thanks.
Mucho mejor, gracias a dios. = Much better, thank God.
Un poco mejor, gracias. = A little better, thanks. (Notice that it is common to say this even if the person is still very sick.)
Gracias, es buen muchacho. = Thank you, he's a good boy.
Gracias, es buena muchacha. = Thank you, she's a good girl.
Ay, mi hijo/hija. Me vuelve loco. = Oh, my son/daughter.

He/She drives me crazy. (If you are female, say, *Me vuelve loca.*)

No puedo creer que sea tan grande. = I can't believe she/he is so grown-up.

If a baby is presented to you, it is proper to make a fuss. Babies are the center of a Latino family's universe, and believe me, what you think is too much gushiness will not seem that way to the family.

¡Ay, qué lindo! = Oh, what a pretty baby! (*linda* = "pretty girl," *lindo* = "pretty boy")

¡Ay, qué gordito! ¡Precioso! = Oh, what a sweetie! Precious! (*Gordita* and *preciosa* for a girl; *gordito/a* is literally "fatty," but it's an endearment, not an insult, in Spanish. How about that for a cultural difference!)

At the end of the day, it's courteous to say a little something about the family:

Saludos a sus padres. = Say hi to your parents.

Espero que su mamá se mejore. = I hope your mother gets better.

Déle a Elena mis felicitaciones. = Give Elena my congratulations.

CHAPTER 13

Past-Tense Verbs

What if you want to talk about something in the past without connecting it to this moment, as you do with the before-now verbs? The simple, past-tense verbs you use in that situation are called the "preterit," which is Latin for "past" or "over with." (See all the Latin you learn when you study Spanish?)

Often the preterit will be accompanied by little bits of information about time, such as *ayer* [yesterday], *anoche* [last night], *anteayer* [day before yesterday], *la semana pasada* [last week], *el año pasado* [last year], *hace dos meses* [two months ago], *hace dos años* [two years ago], *hace un momento* [a momento ago], and *esta mañana* [this morning].

Regular Past-Tense Verbs

To form the preterit verbs, remove the infinitive ending and then add new endings, as you did with the present verbs.

The preterit *-ar* verb endings

-é	-amos
-aste	
-ó	-aron

hablar = hablé, hablaste, habló, hablamos, hablaron
[I spoke, you spoke, he/she/you spoke, we spoke, they/y'all
spoke]

The preterit *-er* and *-ir* verb endings

-í	-imos
-iste	
-ió	-ieron

vivir = viví, viviste, vivió, vivimos, vivieron
[I lived, you lived, he/she/you lived, we lived, they/ya'll
lived]

comer = comí, comiste, comió, comimos, comieron
[I ate, you ate, he/she/you ate, we ate, they/ya'll ate]

How about the weak-kneed verbs? If you look at the stress patterns
explained in chapter 5, you'll see that the weak vowel is protected in
the preterit, because the stress is on the ending. So most, not all, weak-
kneed verbs do not break apart in the preterit:

volver (ue) = volví, volviste, volvió, volvimos, volvieron
[I returned, you returned, he/she/you returned, we returned,
they/ya'll returned]

*entender (ie) = entendí, entendiste, entendió, entendimos,
entendieron*
[I understood, you understood, he/she/you understood,
we understood, they/ya'll understood]

EXERCISE 13-1

Conjugate the following verbs in the preterit.

comprar	vender	abrir
trabajar	volver	añadir
cerrar	perder	reunir
terminar	ver	cubrir
lavar	toser	decidir

Irregular Past-Tense Verbs

Are there irregulars in the preterit? You bet. And one thing about the irregulars in the preterit—they're not fooling around; they're really irregular! Where did that *fui* business come from? Never mind, here are some common verbs that are irregular in the preterit:

> *hacer* = *hice, hiciste, hizo, hicimos, hicieron*
> [I made, you made, he/she/you made, we made, they/ya'll made]

> *decir* = *dije, dijiste, dijo, dijimos, dijero*n
> [I said, you said, he/she/you said, we said, they/ya'll said]

> *ir* = *fui, fuiste, fue, fuimos, fueron*
> [I went, you went, he/she/you went, we went, they/ya'll went]

> *poner* = *puse, pusiste, puso, pusimos, pusieron*
> [I put, you put, he/she/you put, etc.]

> *dar* = *di, diste, dio, dimos, dieron*
> [I gave, you gave, etc.]

> *estar* = *estuve, estuviste, estuvo, estuvimos, estuvieron*
> *ser* = *fui, fuiste, fue, fuimos, fueron* (Yes, this is the same as *ir.*)
> [I was, you were, etc.]

tener = tuve, tuviste, tuvo, tuvimos, tuvieron
[I got or had, etc.]

venir = vine, viniste, vino, vinimos, vinieron
[I came, etc.]

traer = traje, trajiste, trajo, trajimos, trajeron
[I brought, etc.]

EXERCISE 13-2

Write out the preterit conjugations of the irregular verbs shown above. (Writing them out helps ingrain them in your memory.)

These weak-kneed verbs have a weakness in the preterit, but only in the third person:

dormir (ue, u) = dormí, dormiste, durmió, dormimos, durmieron
Another verb patterned like *dormir: morir.*

pedir (i,i) = pedí, pediste, pidió, pedimos, pidieron
Other verbs patterned like *pedir: preferir, medir, servir, repetir, seguir*

EXERCISE 13-3

Write out the conjugations of the weak-kneed verbs above.

EXERCISE 13-4

Fill in the blanks with the appropriate form of the verb in the preterit. Example: *Yo tuve (tener) un problema con el tractor.* [I had a problem with the tractor.]

    1. Alejandro y Felipe _____ (*descornar* = "to dehorn")
        los cabritos ayer.

2. Elías _____ (*descolar* = "to dock") los corderos
   nuevos esta mañana.

3. Yo _____ (aprender) un programa nuevo en el
   taller de computadoras la semana pasada.

4. ¡El precio de la gasolina _____ (subir) otra vez!
   (*otra vez* = "again")

5. Arturo y yo _____ (decidir) no comprar el toro.

6. Yo _____ (cambiar) la dieta de las gallinas, pero
   ellas _____ (preferir) la dieta vieja.

7. El veterinario le _____ (prestar) el manual a usted,
   ¿no? ¿Se lo _____ (*devolver* = "to return" [something
   loaned]) usted a él?

8. Nosotros _____ (hacer) el muesqueo [ear marking]
   ayer todo el día. ¡ _____ (estar) cansados!

9. Rosa y Julio _____ (hacer) todo lo posible, pero
   el cordero _____ (morir).

10. ¡Esas vacas _____ (romper) la cerca otra vez!

EXERCISE 13-5

Change the following phrases to Spanish. Example: "I sheared the
sheep." = *Esquilé las ovejas.*

1. Did you close the gate?
2. Tomasa gave the chicks some pellets.
3. I went to the creek.
4. Did you sterilize the tank?
5. What did the inspector say?
6. Manuel covered the wound with a bandage.
7. Did you bring the disinfectant?
8. The calf coughed a lot last night.
9. We finished late last night. I drank a lot of coffee this morning!
   (*coffee* = "el café")
10. The calf responded well to the antibiotic. It ran to the trough
    this morning with no problem.

Accidents _____

There is a special way of discussing accidents that happen out of the blue. In these cases, you aren't focusing on the culprit or the initiator of the action. You focus instead on saying that it happened to the animal. In this formula, the phrase consists of three parts: *se, le,* and a verb in the past. Example: *Se le rompió la pierna.* (Literally, "the leg broke itself for him." In regular English, "He broke his leg.")

> *¿Qué le pasó?* or *¿Qué le sucedió?* = "What happened (to the animal)?"
> *Se le fracturó la pierna.* = It fractured its leg.
> *Se le infectó la pezuña.* = Its hoof got infected.

Other verbs just use *se* and the preterit:

> *Se tragó un clavo.* = It swallowed a nail.
> *Se cayó en el arroyo.* = It fell in a ditch.
> *Se cortó con un alambre de púas.* = It cut itself on barbed wire.
> *Se electrocutó comiendo el hilo eléctrico.* = It electrocuted itself eating an electrical wire.
> *Se peleó con otro animal.* = It had a fight with another animal.
> *Se embrolló en el alambre de púas.* = It got tangled in the barbed wire.
> *Se atascó en el lodo.* = It got stuck in the mud.

But when you want to identify the perpetrator, don't use *se:*

> *¿Qué le pasó a la vaca?* = What happened to the cow?
> *Le dispararon unos cazadores.* = Some hunters shot it.
> *Le picó una culebra.* = A snake bit it.
> *Le mordió un coyote.* = A coyote bit it.
> *Le atropelló el camión Wal-Mart.* = The Wal-Mart truck ran over it.

EXERCISE 13-6

Change the sentences to Spanish.

1. It swallowed a wire.
2. The foot got infected.
3. It fell in a hole. ("hole in the ground" = *el hoyo*)
4. It cut itself on a nail.
5. It broke its rib.
6. It got stuck in the creek.
7. A dog bit it.
8. The car ran over it.
9. They had a fight.
10. It cut itself on the gate.

CHAPTER 14

Review of Verbs

Feeling a little overwhelmed? Maybe *a lot* overwhelmed? This seems like a good time to stop and review the verbs that you've learned, because you have indeed learned a lot. So far, you've learned the present, infinitive phrases, commands, before-now verbs, and preterit verbs. Let's stop for a moment and try to sort them out into a system.

Take an idea such as "milk the cows." Here are some verb variations on that idea:

I milk the cows every day.
I will milk the cows tomorrow.
I have already milked the cows.
I milked the cows this morning.
Milk the cows! Tell Kevin to milk the cows.

Here are the negative versions of those ideas:

I do not milk the cows every day.
I will not milk the cows tomorrow.
I still have not milked the cows.
I did not milk the cows this morning.
Don't milk the cows! Tell Kevin not to milk the cows.

Now, let's put all those time frames into Spanish:

Ordeño las vacas todos los días.
Voy a ordeñar las vacas mañana.

Ya he ordeñado las vacas.
Ordeñé las vacas esta mañana.
¡Ordeñe las vacas! Dígale a Kevin que ordeñe las vacas.

And the negative forms:

No ordeño las vacas todos los días.
No voy a ordeñar las vacas mañana.
No he ordeñado las vacas todavía.
No ordeñé las vacas esta mañana.
¡No ordeñe las vacas! Dígale a Kevin que no ordeñe las vacas.

Don't forget the infinitive phrases:

I am going to milk the cows tomorrow. = *Voy a ordeñar las vacas mañana.*
I have to milk the cows. = *Tengo que ordeñar las vacas.*
I have just milked the cows. = *Acabo de ordeñar las vacas.*
I want to milk the cows. = *Quiero ordeñar las vacas.*
I can milk the cows. = *Puedo ordeñar las vacas.*
I need to milk the cows. = *Necesito ordeñar las vacas.*
I should milk the cows. = *Debo ordeñar las vacas.*

That's an impressive amount of information, isn't it? So, let's practice it enough that you can feel confident and eager to try it out rather than be overwhelmed. To help, here are some useful words and phrases that indicate time:

present and future time	past time
hoy [today]	ayer [yesterday]
esta noche [tonight]	anoche [last night]
mañana [tomorrow]	esta mañana [this morning]
la semana que viene [next week]	la semana pasada [last week]
este año [this year]	el año pasado [last year]

present and future time	past time
pasado mañana [day after tomorrow]	anteayer [day before yesterday]
más tarde [later]	ya [already]
en dos meses [in two months]	hace dos meses [two months ago]
ahora [now]	hace un momento [a minute ago]
ahora mismo [right now]	hace mucho ya [a while back]

EXERCISE 14-1

Change the following sentences to Spanish.

1. Tomás washes the trailer today. ("to wash" = *lavar*)

Tomás will wash the trailer this afternoon.
Tomás has already washed the trailer.
Tomás washed the trailer this morning.
Tomás, wash the trailer! Tell Tomás to wash the trailer.
Tomás ought to wash the trailer tonight.

2. Today we repair the fence. ("to repair" = *reparar*)

We will repair the fence the day after tomorrow.
We have already repaired the fence.
We repaired the fence yesterday.
It's important that we repair the fence immediately
    ("immediately, right now" = *ahora mismo*).
We have to repair the fence right now.

3. Karen fills the feeder with corn every morning.
    ("to fill" = *llenar*)

Karen filled the feeder yesterday.
Karen has filled the feeder twice this week.
Karen will fill the feeder again tomorrow.
Karen has just filled the feeder.
Karen, fill the feeder please. Tell Karen to fill the feeder.

4. Ann and Carolyn wrote the results in the logbook.
   ("to write" = *escribir*)

Ann and Carolyn have already written the results in the
   logbook.
Ann and Carolyn write the results in the logbook every day
   without fail.
Ann and Carolyn will write the results in the logbook later.
Tell them to write the results in the logbook.
Ann and Carolyn need to write the results in the logbook.

5. I will measure the piglets this afternoon.
   ("to measure" = *medir;* weak-kneed *e* to *i*)

I measured the piglets the day before yesterday.
I want to measure the piglets today.
I have already measured the piglets twice.
Tell Paco to help me.

6. Carl distributes the bales to the pasture.
   ("to distribute" = *repartir*)

It's 6:00, and Carl has already distributed the bales.
Carl distributed the bales to the north pasture.
Carl has to distribute bales today.
Carl, distribute the bales please. Tell Carl to distribute the
   bales to the south pasture.

7. You (informal) prepare the mash well.
   ("to prepare" = *preparar*)

You prepared too much mash yesterday.
You can prepare the mash later.
You have already prepared the mash. Well done!

You don't have to prepare the mash. I can do it.

8. We called the vet. ("to call" = *llamar*)

We have called the vet; he should arrive soon.
We call the vet when there are problems.
We will call the vet tomorrow.
Tell Mr. Kemp to call the vet.

9. The old ram isn't eating well. ("to eat" = *comer*)

The ram ate well last week.
The ram has always eaten well.
The ram needs to eat well.
I think that the ram is sick.

10. The Gómez family sells some calves every year.
    ("to sell" = *vender*)

The Gómez family has sold three calves this year.
The Gómez family sold three calves last year.
The Gómez family will sell four calves next week.
Tell Mr. Gómez to sell me the black calf.

CHAPTER 15

Time and Weather

Telling Time

To tell time in Spanish, we use a three-word formula with the verb *ser*. The first word in the formula is *es* or *son*. The second word is either *la* or *las*. The third word is the number of hours; if it's just one, the first two words are singular. If it's more than one, the first two words are plural:

> *¿Qué hora es?* or *¿Qué horas son?* = "What time is it?"

> 1:00 = *Es la una.*
> 2:00 = *Son las dos.*
> 3:00 = *Son las tres.*
> 4:00 = *Son las cuatro.*

To show the half hour, add *y media,* which means "and a half":

> *¿Qué hora es?*

> 1:30 = *Es la una y media.*
> 5:30 = *Son las cinco y media.*
> 6:30 = *Son las seis y media.*
> 7:30 = *Son las siete y media.*

To show fifteen minutes after, add *y cuarto* [and a fourth] or *y quince* [and fifteen]:

> *¿Qué hora es?*
>
> 1:15 = *Es la una y cuarto* or *Es la una y quince.*
> 8:15 = *Son las ocho y cuarto.*
> 9:15 = *Son las nueve y cuarto.*

To show other minutes past the hour, up to the half hour, just add the number of minutes:

> *¿Qué hora es?*
>
> 1:20 = *Es la una y veinte.*
> 10:18 = *Son las diez y dieciocho.*
> 11:22 = *Son las once y veintidós.*

To show minutes past the half hour, such as 11:40, the official grammar books state that you should say, *"Son las doce menos veinte."* However, in ordinary conversation, Spanish speakers these days tend to say something else. One thing that is increasingly heard is the continuation of the formula stated above:

> 11:40 = *Son las once y cuarenta.*
> 2:50 = *Son las dos y cincuenta.*
> 3:45 = *Son las tres y cuarenta y cinco.*

Some observers attribute this pattern to the influence of English on the Spanish spoken in the United States, Mexico, and Central America. Others attribute it to the growing use of digital watches that don't display the whole clock face, just the numbers with a colon between the hour and minutes.

The other, more common strategy (and the phrase that you should learn) is to say, *Faltan … minutos para la/las …* Literally, "It lacks … minutes for the … hour":

> 11:40 = *Faltan veinte minutos para las doce.*
> 2:50 = *Faltan diez minutos para las tres.*
> 3:45 = *Faltan quince minutos para las cuatro.*
> 12:55 = *Faltan cinco minutos para la una.*

EXERCISE 15-1

Write out the Spanish of the following times. Example: 3:00 = *Son las tres.*

1. 11:45
2. 5:00
3. 6:20
4. 2:30
5. 12:15
6. 12:40
7. 1:25
8. 4:30
9. 8:00
10. 3:15

Time in the Past

To tell time in the past ("It was four o'clock when the inspector arrived"), use *era* instead of *es* and *eran* in place of *son* (*"Eran las cuatro cuando el inspector llegó"*).

When we tell time, we like to add little bits of information like these: *en punto* [on the dot], *más o menos* [more or less], *ya* [already], *de la mañana* [in the morning], and *de la tarde* [in the afternoon]. Numberless times include *el mediodía* [noon], *la medianoche* [midnight], *el amanecer* [dawn], *el anochecer* [nightfall], *tarde* [late], and *temprano* [early].

EXERCISE 15-2

Change the following phrases to Spanish. Example: "It was early when we finished." = *Era temprano cuando terminamos.*

1. It was midnight when we finished.
2. It was 3:00 on the dot when the truck arrived.
3. It was 6:00 in the morning when they began.
4. It was 8:30, more or less, when the cow gave birth.
5. It was already noon when Luz finally returned.

At What Time?

The above ways of telling time are for the circumstances when someone says *¿Qué hora es?* [What time is it?], and they expect you to look at your watch and make a pronouncement. But we also include times in sentences. In these cases, we aren't discussing the time right now; we're discussing when an action will happen. For instance, we can say, "The inspector will arrive at 4:00" at any time leading up to four o'clock. (At four o'clock we say, "He should be here by now. Looks like he's running late.") To include a time in a "nonwatch" sentence, use the phrase *a la/las* ... (at ...):

> *¿A qué hora llega el inspector?* = At what time does the inspector arrive?
> *El inspector va a llegar a las cuatro.* = The inspector is going to arrive at four o'clock.

> *¿A qué hora llegó el inspector?* = At what time did the inspector arrive?
> *El inspector llegó a las cuatro.* = The inspector arrived at four o'clock.

> *¿A qué hora termina usted el trabajo hoy?* = At what time will you finish work today?
> *Tengo que terminar hoy a la una.* = I have to finish today at one o'clock.

> *¿A qué hora terminó usted el trabajo hoy?* = At what time did you finish work today?
> *Tuve que terminar hoy a la una.* = I had to finish today at one o'clock.

> *¿Cuándo vamos a tener más fertilizante?* = When are we going to have more fertilizer?
> *Germán va a recogerlo hoy a las nueve y media.* = Germán is going to pick it up today at nine-thirty.

Germán ya lo recogió a las nueve y media esta mañana. =
Germán already picked it up at nine-thirty this morning.

Answer the following questions with the time indicated. Example:
¿A qué hora terminamos hoy? (5:00) = *Terminamos hoy a las cinco.*
¿A qué hora terminamos ayer? = *Terminamos a las cinco ayer.*

1. ¿A qué hora empieza el ordeño generalmente? (5:00)
   (*generalmente* = "generally")
2. ¿A qué hora empezó el ordeño esta mañana?
   (5:00 on the dot)
3. ¿Cuándo vuelve David? (11:00 more or less)
4. ¿A qué hora volvió David anoche? (11:00 more or less)
5. ¿A qué hora comemos hoy? (12:30)
6. ¿A qué hora comimos ayer? (2:00)
7. ¿A qué hora tiene usted que ir al médico? (9:15)
   (*el médico* = "doctor")
8. ¿A qué hora fue su cita con el médico ayer? (9:15)
   (*la cita* = "appointment")

Weather

Does a day go by when we don't talk about the weather? I suppose
that technically it's *possible* to go for twenty-four whole hours without
mentioning the weather or at least casting an eye on it, but it sure isn't
probable. The truth is, the weather is an important concern for
everyone, and we talk about it a lot in both English and Spanish.

¡Qué lindo día! ¡Qué día más feo! = What a pretty day! What
an ugly day!
¿Qué tiempo hace hoy? = What's the weather like today?
Hace buen tiempo. Hace mal tiempo. = It's nice weather. It's
bad weather.

Hace calor. Hace frío. = It's hot. It's cold.

Hace un calor tremendo. Hace un frío tremendo. = It's awfully hot. It's awfully cold.

¿Va a llover? ¿Va a nevar? = Is it going to rain? Is it going to snow?

Creo que sí. No creo or *Creo que no.* = I think so. I don't think so.

Se dice que va a haber aguacero hoy. = They say that there will be a thundershower today.

Se dice que va a hacer sol hoy. = They say that it will be sunny today.

Parece que va a llover. Parece que no va a llover. = Looks like it's going to rain. Looks like it isn't going to rain.

Ya viene la tormenta. = A storm's coming.

Está nublado. Está medio nublado. = It's cloudy. It's partly cloudy.

Hace viento. Hace mucho viento. = It's windy. It's very windy.

Espero que llueva. Espero que no llueva. = I hope it rains. I hope it doesn't rain.

¿Sintió el trueno? ¿Sintió el relámpago? = Was that thunder? Was that lightning?

Tenemos que terminar antes de que llueva. = We have to finish before it rains.

Vamos a tratar de terminar antes de que llueva. = Let's try to finish before it rains.

Llovió más el año pasado. = It rained more last year.

Ha llovido mucho últimamente. = It's rained a lot recently.

Last year was worse. = *El año pasado fue peor.*

Last year was better. = *El año pasado fue mejor.*

CHAPTER 16

Safety and Hiring

Safety

accidents	los accidentes
antibacterial	el bactericida
apron	el delantal
be careful	tenga cuidado
boots	las botas
careful!	¡cuidado!
danger	peligro
dangerous	peligroso, peligrosa
disinfectant	el desinfectante
emergency exit	la salida de emergencia
emergency number	el número de emergencia
first aid	los primeros auxilios
first aid kit	el botiquín
fungicide	el fungicida
gloves	los guantes
health	la salud
helmet	el casco
mask	la máscara
overalls	el overol

protective glasses, safety glasses	los lentes protectores
safety, security	la seguridad
toxic substance	la sustancia tóxica

Póngase estos guantes para protegerse. = Put on these gloves to protect yourself.

Póngase esta máscara para protegerse. = Put on this mask to protect yourself.

Póngase este delantal. = Put on this apron.

Es importante que se ponga los lentes protectores. = It's important that you put on safety glasses.

Tenga cuidado con esto; es una sustancia tóxica. = Be careful with this; it's a toxic substance.

No queremos accidentes. = We don't want accidents.

CULTURAL NOTE: FOLK MEDICINE

Many people of Hispanic heritage prefer to treat their minor ailments with folk remedies rather than U.S.-style technological medicine. In part, this is because U.S.-style medicine is extremely expensive. It can also be terrifying, with its impersonal stainless steel and hushed corridors. (Now that I think about it, those are the same reasons that some non-Hispanics avoid U.S.-style medicine!)

For minor ailments—colds, headaches, upset stomachs, and so on—many Latinos prefer to drink an herbal tea. There is a rich tradition of herbal remedies in Hispanic culture, and quite a few of them do seem to make the patient feel better. Chamomile tea, for example, seems to help a queasy stomach, and it also helps some people fall asleep at night. You need to keep a well-stocked first-aid kit on hand, of course, but it's a nice gesture to stock some herbal teas as well.

✐ Hiring

La Contratación

address	la dirección
age	la edad
birth date	la fecha de nacimiento
(month/day/year)	(mes/día/año)
contract	el contrato
driver's license number	el número de la
	licencia de manejo
first name	el nombre de pila
insurance	el seguro
last names	los apellidos
marital status	el estado civil
medical exam	el examen médico
phone number	el número de teléfono
signature	la firma
Social Security number	el número de seguro social

Busco alguien que sepa ... = I'm looking for someone who knows how to ...
Busco alguien que sepa ordeñar vacas. = I'm looking for someone who knows how to milk cows.

Busco alguien que pueda ... = I'm looking for someone who can ....
Busco alguien que pueda manejar un tractor. = I'm looking for someone who can drive a tractor.

¿Tiene usted experiencia con ...? = Do you have experience with ... ?
¿Tiene usted experiencia con esquilar las ovejas? = Do you have experience with shearing sheep?

El puesto paga ... dólares la hora. = The job pays ... dollars an hour.

Necesito alguien que pueda trabajar ... días la semana. = I need someone who can work ... days a week.

Venga mañana a las cinco de la mañana, listo para trabajar. = Come tomorrow at five in the morning, ready to work.

Nos vemos mañana a las cinco de la mañana. = We'll see you tomorrow at five in the morning.

El trabajo comienza mañana a las cinco de la mañana. = Work starts at five in the morning.

¿Tiene usted amigos o parientes que también puedan trabajar? = Do you have friends or relatives who can also work?

Dígales que vengan mañana con usted. = Tell them to come tomorrow with you.

CULTURAL NOTE: NEPOTISM

Remember the discussion about the importance of family in chapter 12? In hiring, the traditional family network may work to your advantage. It is common practice in Latin America for relatives to work with each other. The personnel in a restaurant or a store, for instance, may all be related in some way. When you are looking for workers, remember to ask if they have relatives who could sign on too. Workers may feel more loyalty to a job where their relatives are also employed, and thus you may have less turnover of personnel.

CHAPTER 17

Nutrition

Vocabulary

Do you need to learn all of this vocabulary? Probably not. Look for the terms that you use daily, and learn those. For the other terms that you use only once in a while, keep this book on hand and look them up when you need them. And there are some terms that you may never need to know!

additive	el aditivo
amino acid	el aminoácido
amylase	la amilasa
antibiotics	los antibióticos
antioxidant	el antioxidante
ascorbic acid	el ácido ascórbico
ash	la ceniza
bale	la paca
barley	la cebada
beet	la remolacha
Bermuda grass	el pasto bermuda
block	el bloque
bluegrass	el pasto azul

bolus	el bolo
bran	el salvado
cake	la torta
calcium	el calcio
calories	las calorías
carbohydrate	el carbohidrato
carotene	el caroteno
carrier	el vehículo
cellulose	la celulosa
chaff	la cáscara
citric pulp	la pulpa de cítricos
commercial feed	el alimento comercial
concentrate	el concentrado
cooked food	el cocinado
copper	el cobre
cottonseed cake	la torta de algodón
cracked	quebrado, quebrada
crop, harvest	la cosecha
crude fat	la grasa cruda
crude fiber	la fibra cruda
crude protein	la proteína cruda
crumbled food	el alimento en grano
crushed grain	el grano triturado
cud	el bolo alimenticio
dehulled	descascarillada
diet	la dieta
dry matter	la materia seca
enzyme	la enzima
fat	la grasa
fatty acid	el ácido graso
fistula	la fistula
flakes	las hojuelas
flour, meal	la harina
fodder	el forraje, el pienso
fodder crops	las plantas forrajeras
gastric juice	el jugo gástrico

germ	el germen
gluten	el gluten
grain	el grano
to grind	moler
grits	la sémola
ground	molido, molida
hay	el heno
hunger	el hambre
to ingest	ingerir
ingested	ingerido, ingerida
ingredient	el ingrediente
iodine	el yodo
iron	el hierro
lactase	la lactasa
lactic acid	el ácido láctico
lignin	la lignina
lipids	los lípidos
magnesium	el magnesio
manganese	el manganeso
meal, food	el alimento
methane	el metano
minerals	los minerales
mix	la mezcla
to mix	mezclar
molasses	la melaza
niacin	la niacina
nutrients	los nutrientes
nutritional value	el valor nutritivo
oats	la avena
obesity	la obesidad
oil	el aceite
pellets	los pelets
phosphorus	el fósforo
potassium	el potasio
premix	la premezcla
protein	la proteína

rancid	rancio, rancia
ration	la ración
riboflavin	la riboflavina
rolled	rolado, rolada
rye	el centeno
salt	la sal
salt lick, salt block	la salegar, el saladero
scratched	raspado, raspada
sedum	la hierba callera
silage	el ensilaje
sorghum	el sorgo
sorghum silage	el ensilado de sorgo
starch	el almidón
stubble	el rastrojo
straw	la paja; la pajilla *(reproduction)*
Sudan grass	el pasto Sudán
sugars	los azúcares
supplement	el suplemento
thiamin	la tiamina
toasted	tostado, tostada
urea	la urea
vitamin	la vitamina
zinc	el zinc

Some Handy Phrases

What do you give them to eat? = *¿Qué les da de comer?*

We give them hay. = *Les damos el heno.*

We give them sorghum. = *Les damos el sorgo.*

Do you give them vitamins? = *¿Les da vitaminas?*

Yes, and other supplements too. = *Sí, y otros suplementos también.*

Where are the cottonseed cakes? = *¿Dónde están las tortas de algodón?*

They're in the storage barn. = *Están en el almacén.*

The mash consists of a mixture of... = *El puré consiste en una mezcla de...*

Prepare the mash, please. = *Prepare el puré, por favor.*

Add a little more bran. = *Agregue un poco más de salvado.*

Give the sheep the commercial feed. = *Déles a las ovejas el alimento comercial.*

Give them calcium. = *Déles el calcio.*

The old boar, is he eating well? = *El cerdo viejo, ¿come bien?*

The chicks, are they eating well? = *Los pollitos, ¿comen bien?*

Fill the feed trough, please. = *Llene el comedero, por favor.*

Fill the water trough. = *Llene el bebedero.*

Put these salt licks over there. = *Ponga estas salegares allí.*

The barley is running out. = *Se acaba la cebada.*

The barley has run out. (We're out of barley) = *Se acabó la cebada.*

The pellets are running out. = *Se acaban los pelets.*

The pellets have run out. (We're out of pellets) = *Se acabaron los pelets.*

Digestive Organs and Systems

alimentary tract	el tracto alimenticio
digestive tract	el tracto digestivo
monogastric	monogástrico, monogástrica
polygastric	poligástrico, poligástrica
ruminant	el rumiante
rumination	la rumia
abomasum	el abomaso
anus	el ano
cecum	el ciego
cloaca	la cloaca
colon	el colon

duodenum	el duodeno
esophagus	el esófago
gallbladder	la vesícula biliar
gizzard	la molleja
ileum	el íleo
jejunum	el yeyuno
large intestine	el intestino grueso
liver	el hígado
omasum	el omaso
pancreas	el páncreas
rectum	el recto
reticulum	el retículo
rumen	el rumen
small intestine	el intestino delgado
stomach	el estómago

CHAPTER 18

Reproduction

Anatomy

cervix	el cuello uterino
epididymis	el epidídimo
infundibulum	el infundíbulo
mammary gland	la glándula mamaria
ovary	el ovario
oviduct	el oviducto
penis	el pene
prostate	la próstata
scrotum	el escroto
seminal vesicle	la vesícula seminal
teat	la teta, el pezón
testicle	el testículo
udder	la ubre
uterus	el útero
vagina	la vagina
vulva	la vulva

Hormones

estrogen	el estrógeno
follicle-stimulating hormone	la hormona folículo-estimulante, *or* la hormona estimulante del folículo
luteinizing hormone	la hormona luteinizante
oxytocin	la oxitocina
pregnant mare serum (gonadotropin)	la gonadotropina sérica de la yegua preñada
progesterone	la progesterona
prostaglandin	la prostaglandina

The Reproductive Process

artificial insemination	la inseminación artificial
corpus luteum	el cuerpo lúteo
electroejaculation	la electroeyaculación
embryo	el embrión
embryo sexing	el sexado de embriones
embryo splitting	la bipartición de embriones
embryo transfer	la transferencia de embriones
estrus	el estro
fetus	el feto
gestation	la gestación
in vitro fertilization	la fertilización in vitro
lactation	la lactacíon
oocyte	el ovocito
ovulation	la ovulación
palpation	la palpacíon
parturition	el parto
semen	el semen
sperm	el esperma
spermatozoid	el espermatozoide
synchronization of estrus	la sincronización del estro

Instruments and Equipment

canister	la canastilla
cryovial	el criovial
gloves	los guantes
heat patch	el parche detector de calores
liquid nitrogen tank	el tanque de nitrógeno líquido
obstetric chain	la cadena obstétrica
straw	la pajilla

CHAPTER 19

Cattle

Do you want even more vocabulary about cattle? Try using *ganado de carne* or *ganado de leche* as a search term on the Internet. You'll find lots of sites, announcements, and discussions in Spanish. Also, ask your local university or cooperative extension agency if they have bulletins or other materials in Spanish.

Animals and People

beef cattle	el ganado de carne
breed	la raza
Brown Swiss breed	la raza pardo suiza
bull	el toro
calf	el ternero, el becerro
cattle	el ganado
cow	la vaca
cowman, cowboy	el vaquero
cow woman, cowgirl	la vaquera
dairy cattle	el ganado de leche
dry cow	la vaca seca
feedlot cattle	el ganado estabulado
grazing cattle	el ganado en pastoreo

heifer	la vaquilla, la novilla
herd	el rebaño, el hato, el ganado
milker	el ordeñador, la ordeñadora
Milking Shorthorn	la raza cuernos cortos lechera
ox	el buey
spring heifer	la vaquilla a parto
steer	el torete, el novillo
yearling	el añal

Buildings and Installations

box stall	el cubículo
building for processing or selling milk	la lechería
calf hutch	la becerrera
chute	la manga, la rampa
dark box	el cajón
dipping vat	el baño de inmersión
elevated stall	el corral elevado
feedlot	el corral de engorda
foot bath	el pediluvio
free stall	el estabulado libre
loading ramp	la rampa de carga
lockup; cage crate; cage chute	la trampa ajustable
milking parlor	la sala de ordeño
milking system	el sistema de ordeño
squeeze chute	la prensa, la trampa
weighing crate; scales	la báscula

Equipment and Other Terms

branding	el marcaje
branding iron	el hierro a marcar
ear tag	el arete

electric clippers	la esquiladora
manure	el estiércol
mastitis test	la prueba de mastitis
neck chain; collar	el collar
nipple bottle	el biberón
nose tongs	el nariguero
rope halter	el freno
tattoo	el tatuaje
teat cup	la pezonera

Actions

to brand	marcar
to buy	comprar
to charge, assail	embestir
to dehorn	descornar (ue)
to examine	examinar
to feed	dar de comer
to milk	ordeñar
to moo	mugir
to ruminate	rumiar
to sell	vender
to separate	separar

CHAPTER 20

Sheep and Goats

Many terms used in raising sheep and goats are also used in raising cattle, so terms listed in chapter 19 won't be repeated here. Try using *ovejas* or *cabras* as a search term on the Internet. Also ask your local university or cooperative extension agency if they have bulletins or other materials in Spanish. In Latin America, the extension agencies in Argentina have some very useful bulletins.

Animals

buck	el macho cabrío
doe	la cabra, la cabra hembra
ewe	la cabra, la oveja hembra
fleece	el vellón
flock	el rebaño
goat	la cabra
kid	el cabrito, la cabrita
lamb	el cordero, la cordera
pelt	la piel, el cuero
ram	el carnero
sheep	la oveja, las ovejas
wool	la lana

Equipment and Actions _____

to bleat	balar
dehorning	el descornado
disbudding	el desbotonado
to dock	descolar
docking	el descolado
emasculator	el emasculador
shear	esquilar
shearing facilities	las instalaciones de esquilar
shearing machine	la esquiladora
shearing shed	la muda
sheep foot trimmers	el cortapezuñas
sheep pen, fold	el redil
sorting shunt	la manga separadora

CHAPTER 21

Swine

Check the previous two chapters for vocabulary that is useful for swine raising too. On the Internet, try using *cerdos* or *puerco* as search terms. Consult your local university or cooperative extension agency about bulletins or other materials in Spanish.

Industry and Animals

barrow	el cerdo castrado
boar	el cerdo, el verraco
finishing swine	el cerdo en finalización
gilt	la cerda de reemplazo
growing swine	el cerdo en crecimiento
hog	el porcino
pig	el cerdo
piglet; feeder pig	el lechón, la lechona
pork	el puerco
sow	la cerda, el vientre
swine industry	la industria porcina
weaned swine	el cerdo destetado

Equipment and Actions

back fat determination	la determinación de la grasa dorsal
breeding system	el sistema de reproducción
clipping of the needle teeth	el descolmillado
ear notching	el muesqueo
farrowing	el parto
farrowing crate	la jaula de maternidad
farrowing unit	la maternidad
growing-finishing unit	la unidad de crecimiento-finalización
hog snare	el asa trompas
iron shot	la inyección de hierro
manure pump	la bomba para lodos
manure separator	el separador de estiércol
mating area	el área de monta
navel cord care	el cuidado del cordón umbilical
pigsty	la pocilga
shade	la sombra
slotted floor system	el sistema de piso rasurado
Specific Pathogen-Free (SPF) Program	el program libre de patógenos específicos
tail docking	el descolado
ultrasonic probe	la sonda de ultrasonido
wallow	el revolcadero
weaning unit	la unidad de destete

22

Poultry

There's an increasing amount of useful material about poultry in Spanish on the Internet; try using *avicultura* as a search term. Also, ask your university or cooperative extension agency about Spanish-language bulletins.

Industry, Animals, and People

broiler	el pollo de engorda
capon	el capón
chick	el pollito, la pollita
egg	el huevo
hen	la gallina
layer parent stock	el reproductor de postura
laying hen	la gallina de postura
poultry dealer	el pollero
poultry farming	la avicultura
poultry industry	la industria avícola
pullet	el pollo, la polla
replacement pullet	la polla de reemplazo
roaster	el pollo para asar

Equipment and Actions ────────────────────

aviary	el aviario
bedding	la cama
brooder	la gallina clueca
to candle	mirar a trasluz
controlled environment	el ambiente controlado
coop	la caseta
debeaking	el despicado
dewattling	el desbarbillado
droppings	las heces
dubbing	el descrestado
to hatch	eclosionar
incubator	la incubadora
to lay	poner (huevos)
laying cage	la jaula de postura
leg band	el anillo
nest	el nido
perch	la percha
photo period	el foto período
to pluck	desplumar
plumage	el plumaje
straw litter	la cama
wing badge, wing tag	el arete de la ala

Answer Key to
Exercises
and
Dictionary

Answer Key to Exercises

1-1

1. alfalfa
2. buche
3. corral
4. celo
5. desinfectar
6. ensilaje
7. fiebre
8. garrapata
9. Geraldo
10. heno
11. inseminar
12. joroba
13. leche
14. mastitis
15. novillo
16. oveja
17. pasto
18. quiste
19. rumen
20. sangre
21. ternero
22. ubre
23. vaquilla
24. yodo
25. zanahoria

2-1

1. la torta
2. el alimento
3. el estómago
4. la enfermedad
5. el camión
6. la reproducción
7. la alfalfa
8. el ensilaje
9. la influenza
10. el problema
11. la gestación
12. el hocico
13. el escroto
14. la bronquitis
15. el separador

2-2

1. un cerdo
2. una epidemia
3. un animal
4. un cordero
5. una garrapata
6. una piara
7. un sistema
8. una granja
9. un baño
10. una incubadora

2-3

1. las ubres
2. los partos
3. unas pocilgas
4. unos frenos
5. los biberones
6. unos vaqueros
7. las esquiladoras
8. unas gallinas
9. los tractores
10. las jaulas
11. unas palas
12. unos minerales
13. los trinchetes
14. las enzimas
15. unos ingredientes

3-1

1. la cerda blanca
2. una gallina nueva
3. el becerro (*or* ternero) recién nacido
4. la cabrita parda
5. un toro viejo
6. la oveja preñada
7. un verraco (*or* cerdo) grande
8. el gallo negro
9. el carnero pequeño (*or* chico)
10. una vaca roja

3-2

1. las cerdas blancas
2. unas gallinas nuevas
3. los becerros (*or* terneros) recién nacidos
4. las cabritas pardas
5. unos toros viejos
6. las ovejas preñadas
7. unos verracos (*or* cerdos) grandes
8. los gallos negros

9. los carneros pequeños (*or* chicos)
10. unas vacas rojas

3-3

1. seis becerros (*or* terneros)
2. pocas vacas
3. muchas ovejas
4. ciento ochenta y dos pollitos
5. diecisiete cordero
6. doce cabras
7. veinticuatro lechones
8. muchas gallinas
9. quince toros
10. cien cerdos

3-4

1. seis becerros (*or* terneros) nuevos
2. pocas vacas nuevas
3. muchas ovejas nuevas
4. ciento ochenta y dos pollitos nuevos
5. diecisiete corderos nuevos
6. doce cabras nuevas
7. veinticuatro lechones nuevos
8. muchas gallinas nuevas
9. quince toros nuevos
10. cien cerdos nuevos

3-5

1. esta cerda blanca
2. esa gallina nueva
3. ese becerro (*or* ternero) recién nacido
4. aquella cabrita parda
5. ese toro viejo
6. esta oveja preñada
7. aquel verraco (*or* cerdo) grande
8. este gallo negro

9. ese carnero pequeño (*or* chico)
10. aquella vaca roja

3-6

1. estas cerdas blancas
2. esas gallinas nuevas
3. esos becerros (*or* terneros) recién nacidos
4. aquellas cabritas pardas
5. esos toros viejos
6. estas ovejas preñadas
7. aquellos verracos (*or* cerdos) grandes
8. estos gallos negros
9. esos carneros pequeños (*or* chicos)
10. aquellas vacas rojas

3-7

1. mi granja lechera
2. su granja (*or* finca)
3. nuestra puerta
4. su cerca
5. su tanque de agua
6. su rancho
7. nuestro camino

3-8

1. mis granjas lecheras
2. sus granjas *or* sus fincas
3. nuestras puertas
4. sus cercas
5. sus tanques de agua
6. sus ranchos
7. nuestros caminos

4-1

-ar verbs
yo ordeño, tú ordeñas, él/ella/usted ordeña, nosotros ordeñamos, ellos/ellas/ustedes ordeñan

yo cambio, tú cambias, él/ella/usted cambia, nosotros cambiamos, ellos/ellas/ustedes cambian
reviso, revisas, revisa, revisamos, revisan
lavo, lavas, lava, lavamos, lavan
cuido, cuidas, cuida, cuidamos, cuidan
etc.

-er verbs
corro, corres, corre, corremos, corren
bebo, bebes, bebe, bebemos, beben
aprendo, aprendes, aprende, aprendemos, aprenden
etc.

-ir verbs
abro, abres, abre, abrimos, abren
recibo, recibes, recibe, recibimos, reciben
escribo, escribes, escribe, escribimos, escriben
etc.

4-2

1. él lava
2. nosotros esquilamos
3. ellos escriben
4. ustedes deben
5. ella revisa
6. yo recibo
7. usted cree
8. Pedro agrega (*or* añade)
9. la vaca tose
10. Juanita cuida
11. Juan y Ramón abren
12. María y yo dependemos
13. yo limpio
14. tú cambias
15. Manuel y Lupe ordeñan
16. Carlos y yo terminamos

17. los lechones corren
18. el becerro (*or* el ternero)
    consume
19. usted repara
20. el precio sube
21. yo comprendo

5-1

entiendo, entiendes, entiende,
   entendemos, entienden
comienzo, comienzas, comienza,
   comenzamos, comienzan
recomiendo, recomiendas,
   recomienda, recomendamos,
   recomiendan
pierdo, pierdes, pierde,
   perdemos, pierden
puedo, puedes, puede, podemos,
   pueden
cuesto, cuestas, cuesta, costamos,
   cuestan
duermo, duermes, duerme,
   dormimos, duermen
cuento, cuentas, cuenta,
   contamos, cuentan
mido, mides, mide, medimos,
   miden
sirvo, sirves, sirve, servimos, sirven
repito, repites, repite, repetimos,
   repiten
rindo, rindes, rinde, rendimos,
   rinden

5-2

1. las gallinas duermen
2. nosotros dormimos
3. el veterinario (*or* la
   veterinaria) recomienda
4. Pablo y Norberto pueden
5. esta cerda cuesta
6. ese toro mide
7. usted entiende
8. esta vaca rinde

9. Tomás y yo contamos
10. tú pierdes
11. este restaurante sirve
12. la feria comienza
13. el capataz (*or* la capataz *or*
    el *or* la mayordomo) y la
    inspectora (*or* el inspector)
    repiten
14. el capataz (*or* la capataz *or* el *or*
    la mayordomo) y yo repetimos

5-3

1. las gallinas no duermen
2. nosotros no dormimos
3. el veterinario (*or* la veterinaria)
   no recomienda
4. Pablo y Norberto no pueden
5. esta cerda no cuesta
6. ese toro no mide
7. usted no entiende
8. esta vaca no rinde
9. Tomás y yo no contamos
10. tú no pierdes
11. este restaurante no sirve
12. la feria no comienza
13. el capataz (*or* la capataz, *or* el *or*
    la mayordomo) y la inspectora
    (*or* el inspector) no repiten
14. el capataz (*or* la capataz, *or*
    el *or* la mayordomo) y yo no
    repetimos

5-4

1. La combinada anda bien.
2. ¡La empacadora no anda mal!
3. El tractor no anda bien.
4. Las picadoras funcionan bien.
5. Las cosechadoras andan bien
6. Las camionetas andan bien.
7. El montacargas no funciona
   bien.
8. El mezclador funciona mal.

6-1

1. Hay una venta en Omaha.
2. Estas gallinas están enfermas.
3. Este toro es peligroso.
4. El ganado (*or* el hato, el rebaño, *or* la piara) va al arroyo.
5. Yo tengo mucho trabajo.
6. ¡Estamos cansados!
7. Esa oveja es una Merino.
8. Hay salegares (*or* saladeros) para las cabras.
9. Los lechones tienen suficiente peso.
10. Usted va en la camioneta.

6-2

1. No hay una venta en Omaha.
2. Estas gallinas no están enfermas.
3. Este toro no es peligroso.
4. El ganado (*or* el hato, el rebaño, *or* la piara) no va al arroyo.
5. Yo no tengo mucho trabajo.
6. ¡No estamos cansados!
7. Esa oveja no es una Merino.
8. No hay salegares (*or* saladeros) para las cabras.
9. Los lechones no tienen suficiente peso.
10. Usted no va en la camioneta. Usted va en el camión.

6-3

1. Pablo trae el remolque.
2. Yo traigo el remolque.
3. Jessie y Ray salen tarde.
4. Salgo tarde.
5. Mis amigos no conocen a los García. (*for now, don't worry about the* "a")
6. No conozco a los García.

7. Las vacas vienen despacio al establo.
8. Vengo despacio al establo.
9. Los inspectores dicen que no hay problema.
10. Yo digo que no hay problema.
11. Hacemos nuestros quehaceres.
12. Hago mis quehaceres.
13. Ustedes ponen el heno en el pastizal.
14. Yo pongo el heno en el pastizal.
15. Las ovejas saben que comen pronto.
16. ¡Sé que como pronto!

7-1

1. Tengo que comprar un antibiótico.

Quiero comprar un antibiótico.
Puedo comprar un antibiótico.
Voy a comprar un antibiótico.
Debo comprar un antibiótico.
Acabo de comprar un antibiótico.
Necesito comprar un antibiótico.

2. Debemos vender unos becerros (*or* terneros).

Acabamos de vender unos becerros.
Necesitamos vender unos becerros.
Queremos vender unos becerros.
Podemos vender unos becerros.
Vamos a vender unos becerros.
Tenemos que vender unos becerros.

3. Tienen que entregar el mijo (*or* el millo) hoy.

Van a entregar el mijo hoy.
Necesitan entregar el mijo hoy.
Pueden entregar el mijo hoy.
Acaban de entregar el mijo hoy.
Quieren entregar el mijo hoy.
Deben entregar el mijo hoy.

4. El veterinario quiere
inspeccionar el ganado.

El veterinario acaba de
inspeccionar el ganado.
El veterinario debe inspeccionar
el ganado.
El veterinario va a inspeccionar
el ganado.
El veterinario tiene que
inspeccionar el ganado.
El veterinario necesita
inspeccionar el ganado.
El veterinario puede inspeccionar
el ganado.
El veterinario sabe inspeccionar
el ganado.

5. Usted puede reparar la cerca.

Usted debe reparar la cerca.
Usted va a reparar la cerca.
Usted quiere reparar la cerca.
Usted acaba de reparar la cerca.
Usted tiene que reparar la cerca.
Usted necesita reparar la cerca.
Usted sabe reparar la cerca.

6. No voy a pagar ese precio.

No quiero pagar ese precio.
No tengo que pagar ese precio.
No necesito pagar ese precio.
No debo pagar ese precio.
No puedo pagar ese precio.

7-2

1. ¿Comen las gallinas mucho
sorgo?
2. ¿Rinden las cabras mucha
leche?
3. ¿Puede usted terminar temprano?
4. ¿Son los becerros (*or* terneros)
mansos?

5. ¿Prefieren ustedes las vitaminas
orgánicas?

7-3

1. ¿Cuando llega la veterinaria
(*or* el veterinario)?
2. ¿Dónde debo poner los porcinos
(*or* los cerdos) nuevos?
3. ¿Cuánta leche rinde esta vaca?
4. ¿Cómo responde el ganado a
las tortas de algodón?
5. ¿Cuántas pacas necesita usted?

7-4

1. ¿Quién sabe? Su camioneta
está descompuesta.
2. No sé. ¿Quizás en el pastizal
del norte?
3. No estoy segura (*or* seguro).
Camareno tiene la bitácora.
4. Creo que prefieren la alfalfa.
5. No tengo idea. Quizás tres o
cuatro.

8-1

1. Carlos le da el maíz al cerdo.
2. María le da las vitaminas a la
gallina.
3. Ramón le da los suplementos
a la oveja.
4. Pablo y yo le damos el calcio a
la vaca.
5. Francisco y Martín le dan el
heno al toro.

8-2

1. Carlos le da el maíz.
2. María le da las vitaminas.
3. Ramón le da los suplementos.
4. Pablo y yo le damos el calcio.
5. Francisco y Martín le dan el heno.

8-3

1. Carlos les da el maíz.
2. María les da las vitaminas.
3. Ramón les da los suplementos.
4. Pablo y yo les damos el calcio.
5. Francisco y Martín les dan el heno.

8-4

1. Jaime nos da el informe.
2. Jaime me da el informe.
3. Jaime les da el informe.
4. Jaime te da el informe.
5. Jaime les da el informe a ustedes.
6. Jaime nos da el informe a Hernán y a mí.
7. Jaime le da el informe a Karen.
8. Jaime les da el informe a Hernán y Karen.

8-5

1. Yo le compro rosas a Mamá.
2. Carmen le envía el cheque al vendedor.
3. El señor Jones me vende la avena.
4. Nina les muestra el rancho a los socios del club FFA.
5. Ustedes les dan sus raciones a las gallinas.
6. Miguel y yo les cortamos las uñas a los cerditos.
7. El señor Hernández nos esquila la lana.
8. Usted le presta su navaja a Mario.
9. El inspector le escribe su informe a usted.
10. Nosotros le entregamos las cuentas a la contadora.

9-1

1. Manuel milks the cow.
2. Pablo and Ramón shear the sheep.
3. We unload the bales.
4. They want to buy a new trailer.
5. Do you have the shovel?
6. We clean the stalls every day.
7. You weigh the lambs often.
8. You should read the instructions.
9. The cows break the fence.
10. I sterilize the equipment.

9-2

1. Manuel ordeña la vaca.
2. Pablo y Ramón esquilan las ovejas.
3. Descargamos las pacas.
4. Quieren comprar un remolque nuevo.
5. ¿Tiene usted la pala?
6. Limpiamos los pesebres todos los días.
7. Usted pesa los corderos a menudo.
8. Usted debe leer las instrucciones.
9. Las vacas rompen la cerca.
10. Esterilizo el equipo.

9-3

1. Manuel la ordeña.
2. Pablo y Ramón las esquilan.
3. Las descargamos.
4. Quieren comprarlo. *Or,* Lo quieren comprar.
5. ¿La tiene usted?
6. Los limpiamos todos los días.
7. Usted los pesa a menudo.
8. Usted debe leerlas. *Or,* Usted las debe leer.

9. Las vacas la rompen.
10. Lo esterilizo.

9-4

1. Sí, lo vendo.
2. Sí, la veo.
3. Sí, queremos organizarla. *Or,* Sí, la queremos organizar.
4. Sí, los conozco.
5. Sí, puedo tatuarlas. *Or,* Sí las puedo tatuar.
6. Sí, los tenemos todavía.
7. Ustedes deben descargarlo allí. *Or,* Ustedes lo deben descargar allí.
8. Sí, las busco.
9. Sí, lo necesitamos.
10. Sí, lo hablo.

9-5

1. No, no lo vendo.
2. No, no la veo.
3. No, no queremos organizarla. *Or,* No, no la queremos organizar.
4. No, no los conozco.
5. No, no puedo tatuarlas. *Or,* No, no las puedo tatuar.
6. No, ya no los tenemos. (*Todavía* usually becomes *ya* in negative sentences.)
7. Ustedes no deben descargarlo allí. *Or,* Ustedes no lo deben descargar allí.
8. No, no las busco.
9. No, no lo necesitamos.
10. No, no lo hablo.

10-1

1. limpie, no limpie, limpien, no limpien
2. traiga, no traiga, traigan, no traigan
3. cubra, no cubra, cubran, no cubran
4. repare, no repare, reparen, no reparen
5. ponga, no ponga, pongan, no pongan
6. abra, no abra, abran, no abran
7. esterilice, no esterilice, esterilicen, no esterilicen (When z is followed by e or i, it becomes c, but the sound doesn't change.)
8. trabaje, no trabaje, trabajen, no trabajen
9. suba, no suba, suban, no suban
10. reúna, no reúna, reúnan, no reúnan
11. haga, no haga, hagan, no hagan
12. cierre, no cierre, cierren, no cierren
13. mida, no mida, midan, no midan
14. corte, no corte, corten, no corten
15. prepare, no prepare, preparen, no preparen

10-2

1. Limpie el pesebre.
2. Repare la ordeñadora.
3. Traiga la soga.
4. Añada más cebada. *Or,* Agregue más cebada.
5. Vaya al establo.
6. Inspeccione las pezuñas (*or* los cascos).
7. Vuelva mañana.
8. Cuente los corderos.
9. Abra la puerta.
10. Cierre la puerta.

10-3

1. No limpie el pesebre.
2. No repare la ordeñadora.
3. No traiga la soga.
4. No añada más cebada. *Or,* No agregue más cebada.
5. No vaya al establo.
6. No inspeccione las pezuñas (*or* los cascos).
7. No vuelva mañana.
8. No cuente los corderos.
9. No abra la puerta.
10. No cierre la puerta.

11-1

1. esquile la lana, no esquile la lana
2. tatúele la oreja al carnero, no le tatúe la oreja al carnero
3. cierre la puerta, no cierre la puerta
4. termine los quehaceres, no termine los quehaceres
5. préstele la camioneta a Keith, no le preste la camioneta a Keith
6. lave el suelo, no lave el suelo
7. revise las llantas, no revise las llantas
8. repártales el alambre a las trabajadores, no les reparta el alambre a los trabajadores
9. déles el antibiótico a los becerros (*or* terneros), no les dé el antibiótico a los becerros
10. rompa la botella, no rompa la botella

11-2

1. Préstele el rastrillo. No le preste el rastrillo. Présteselo. No se lo preste.

2. Déme la manguera. No me dé la manguera. Démela. No me la dé.
3. Déle las llaves. No le dé las llaves. Déselas. No se las dé.
4. Tráiganos la carretilla. No nos traiga la carretilla. Tráiganosla. No nos la traiga.
5. Cámbieles la cama a las ovejas. No les cambie la cama a las ovejas. Cámbiesela. No se la cambie.
6. Muéstrele la bitácora. No le muestre la bitácora. Múestresela. No se la muestre.
7. Véndales el remolque. No les venda el remolque. Véndaselo. No se lo venda.
8. Envíele los informes. No le envíe los informes. Envíeselos. No se los envíe.
9. Díganos el chiste. No nos diga el chiste. Díganoslo. No nos lo diga.
10. Présteme un dólar. No me preste un dólar. Préstemelo. No me lo preste.

11-3

1. Dígale a Jack que cierre la puerta.
2. Dígale a Jack que no cierre la puerta.
3. Dígale que lave el camión.
4. Dígale que no lave el camión.
5. Dígale a Lupe que compre más ungüento.
6. Dígale a Lupe que no compre más ungüento.
7. Dígale que me traiga una llave.
8. Dígale que no me traiga una llave.

9. Dígales a Miguel y Arón que me ayuden.
10. Dígales que me ayuden.

11-4

1. Prefiero que limpie el tanque. *Or,* Sugiero que limpie el tanque. *Or,* Es necesario que limpie el tanque. *Or,* Es importante que limpie el tanque.
2. Es necesario que añada agua al bebedero.
3. Sugiero que compre gasolina para la camioneta.
4. Es importante que tenga cuidado con los corderos recién nacidos.
5. Prefiero que cuide de la vaca enferma.
6. Es necesario que trabaje más rápido.
7. Es importante que vaya a la clínica.
8. Sugiero que escriba las notas en la bitácora.
9. Prefiero que lo lave con el desinfectante.
10. Sugiero que separe las gallinas menos productivas.
11. Es importante que examine las patas.
12. Prefiero que los ponga en el corral.
13. Sugiero que los mueva a otro pastizal.
14. Es necesario que corte las alas.
15. Sugiero que los acaricie.

12-1

-ar verbs
he lavado, has lavado, ha lavado, hemos lavado, han lavado

he reparado, has reparado, ha reparado, hemos reparado, han reparado
he terminado, has terminado, ha terminado, hemos terminado, han terminado
etc.

-er verbs
he comido, has comido, ha comido, hemos comido, han comido
he traído, has traído, ha traído, hemos traído, han traído
he leído, has leído, ha leído, hemos leído, han leído
etc.

-ir verbs
he venido, has venido, ha venido, hemos venido, han venido
he repartido, has repartido, ha repartido, hemos repartido, han repartido
he recibido, has recibido, ha recibido, hemos recibido, han recibido
etc.

12-2

he hecho, has hecho, ha hecho, hemos hecho, han hecho
he dicho, has dicho, ha dicho, hemos dicho, han dicho
he abierto, has abierto, ha abierto, hemos abierto, han abierto
he cubierto, has cubierto, ha cubierto, hemos cubierto, han cubierto
he escrito, has escrito, ha escrito, hemos escrito, han escrito
he muerto, has muerto, ha muerto, hemos muerto, han muerto

he roto, has roto, ha roto, hemos
roto, han roto
he visto, has visto, ha visto,
hemos visto, han visto
he vuelto, has vuelto, ha vuelto,
hemos vuelto, han vuelto
he puesto, has puesto, ha puesto,
hemos puesto, han puesto

12-3 _____
1. ha sido
2. ha funcionado
3. han progresado
4. ha consumido
5. Ha pesado
6. he hecho
7. han puesto
8. he registrado
9. hemos comprado, ha
   examinado, ha prometido

✐ **12-4** _____

1. Antonio ha vendido seis
   vaquillas.
2. ¡Creo que han dormido tarde!
3. Eduardo ha separado los
   becerros (*or* terneros) para
   el marcaje.
4. ¿Ya ha limpiado usted la
   maquinaria? *Or,* ¿Ha limpiado
   usted la maquinaria ya? (Words
   such as *ya, todavía,* or *finalmente*
   can go before the verb or at
   the end of the sentence.)
5. Ya no he terminado el informe.
   ¡No lo he comenzado!
6. Luisa ya ha salido.
7. No hemos podido reparar la
   descremadora.
8. La oveja vieja ha muerto.
9. La veterinaria (*or,* el veterinario)
   ha recomendado más calcio.
   ¿Lo ha comprado ya?

10. ¿Ha visto usted mis llaves?
11. El camión con el maíz ha
    llegado finalmente.
12. ¿Ya ha vuelto José?
13. He leído las instrucciones,
    pero no las he entendido.
14. El precio siempre ha subido.
15. Esta vaca no ha rendido tanta
    leche como había esperado.

13-1 _____

-ar verbs
compré, compraste, compró,
   compramos, compraron
trabajé, trabajaste, trabajó,
   trabajamos, trabajaron
etc.

-er verbs
vendí, vendiste, vendió,
   vendimos, vendieron
volví, volviste, volvió,
   volvimos, volvieron
etc.

-ir verbs
abrí, abriste, abrió, abrimos,
   abrieron
añadí, añadiste, añadió,
   añadimos, añadieron
etc.

13-3 _____

morí, moriste, murió, morimos,
   murieron
preferí, preferiste, prefirió,
   preferimos, prefirieron
medí, mediste, midió, medimos,
   midieron
serví, serviste, sirvió, servimos,
   sirvieron
repetí, repetiste, repitió,
   repetimos, repitieron

seguí, seguiste, siguió, seguimos,
   siguieron

13-4 _____

1. descornaron
2. descoló
3. aprendí
4. subió
5. decidimos
6. cambié, prefirieron
7. prestó, devolvió
8. hicimos, estuvimos
9. hicieron, murió
10. rompieron

13-5 _____

1. ¿Cerró usted la puerta?
2. Tomasa le dio unos pelets a los pollitos.
3. Fui al arroyo.
4. ¿Esterilizó usted el tanque?
5. ¿Qué dijo el inspector?
6. Manuel cubrió la herida con un vendaje.
7. ¿Trajo usted el desinfectante?
8. El becerro (*or* ternero) tosió mucho anoche.
9. Terminamos tarde anoche. ¡Bebí mucho café esta mañana!
10. El becerro (*or* ternero) respondió bien al antibiótico. Corrió al comedero esta mañana sin problema.

13-6 _____

1. Se tragó un hilo (*or* alambre).
2. Se le infectó la pata.
3. Se cayó en un hoyo.
4. Se cortó con un clavo.
5. Se le rompió la costilla.
6. Se atascó en el arroyo.

7. Le mordió un perro.
8. Le atropelló el auto.
9. Se pelearon.
10. Se cortó con la puerta.

14-1 _____

1. Tomás lava el remolque hoy.

Tomás va a lavar el remolque esta tarde.

Tomás ya ha lavado el remolque.

Tomás lavó el remolque esta mañana.

Tomás, ¡lave el remolque! Dígale a Tomás que lave el remolque.

Tomás debe lavar el remolque esta noche.

2. Hoy reparamos la cerca. Or, Reparamos la cerca hoy.

Vamos a reparar la cerca pasado mañana.

Ya hemos reparado la cerca.

Reparamos la cerca ayer.

Es importante que reparemos la cerca ahora mismo.

Tenemos que reparar la cerca ahora mismo.

3. Karen llena el comedero con maíz todas las mañanas.

Karen llenó el comedero ayer.

Karen ha llenado el comedero dos veces esta semana.

Karen va a llenar el comedero otra vez mañana.

Karen acaba de llenar el comedero.

Karen, llene el comedero, por favor. Dígale a Karen que llene el comedero.

4. Ann y Carolyn escribieron los resultados en la bitácora.

Ann y Carolyn ya han escrito los resultados en la bitácora.

Ann y Carolyn escriben los resultados en la bitácora todos los días sin falta.

Ann y Carolyn van a escribir los resultados en la bitácora más tarde.

Dígales que escriban los resultados en la bitácora.

Ann y Carolyn necesitan escribir los resultados en la bitácora.

5. Voy a medir los cerditos (or los lechones) esta tarde.

Medí los cerditos anteayer.

Quiero medir los cerditos hoy.

Ya he medido los cerditos dos veces.

Dígale a Paco que me ayude.

6. Carl reparte las pacas al pastizal.

Son las seis, y Carl ya ha repartido las pacas.

Carl repartió las pacas al pastizal del norte.

Carl tiene que repartir las pacas hoy.

Carl, reparta las pacas, por favor.

Dígale a Carl que reparta las pacas al pastizal del sur.

7. Preparas el puré bien.

Preparaste demasiado puré ayer.

Puedes preparar el puré más tarde.

Ya has preparado el puré. ¡Bien hecho!

No tienes que preparar el puré. Yo puedo hacerlo.

8. Llamamos al veterinario.

Hemos llamado al veterinario; debe llegar pronto.

Llamamos al veterinario cuando hay problemas.

Vamos a llamar al veterinario mañana.

Dígale al señor Kemp que llame al veterinario.

9. El carnero viejo no come bien.

El carnero comió bien la semana pasada.

El carnero siempre ha comido bien.

El carnero necesita comer bien.

Creo que el carnero está enfermo.

10. Los Gómez venden unos becerros (or terneros) todos los años.

Los Gómez han vendido tres becerros este año.

Los Gómez vendieron tres becerros el año pasado.

Los Gómez van a vender cuatro becerros la semana que viene.

Dígale al señor Gómez que me venda el becerro negro.

15-1

1. Faltan quince para las doce.
2. Son las cinco.
3. Son las seis y veinte.
4. Son las dos y media.
5. Son las doce y quince.
6. Faltan veinte para la una.
7. Es la una y veinticinco.
8. Son las cuatro y media.
9. Son las ocho.
10. Son las tres y quince.

15-2

1. Era la medianoche cuando terminamos.
2. Eran las tres en punto cuando el camión llegó.

3. Eran las seis de la mañana cuando comenzaron.
4. Eran las ocho y media, más o menos, cuando la vaca parió.
5. Ya era el mediodía cuando Luz finalmente volvió.

🖉 **15-3** _____

1. Empieza a las cinco.
2. Empezó a las cinco en punto.

3. Vuelve a las once, más o menos.
4. Volvió a las once, más o menos.
5. Comemos a las doce y media.
6. Comimos a las dos ayer.
7. Tengo que ir a las nueve y quince.
8. Fue a las nueve y quince.

Dictionary of English and Spanish Terms

The following dictionary does not divide the English and Spanish terms into two separate sections, in the way that most dictionaries are arranged. Instead, the terms are listed together, so that you can quickly find the word you're looking for.

Note: when a verb is followed by vowels in parentheses, that means that the verb is weak-kneed. Please see chapters 5 and 13 for details.

A _____
a—to; (with time) at; when *a* is next to *el,* they combine to form *al*
a little—*un poco*
a lot—*mucho*
a menudo—often
a veces—sometimes
abierto, abierta—open; *la puerta está abierta*—the gate is open
able, be able to—*poder (ue)*
abomaso, el—abomasum
abomasum—*el abomaso*
abril—April

abrir—to open
absorb—*absorber*
absorber—to absorb
acá—here; more informal and conversational than *aquí*
acabar—to have just (done something); *acabo de limpiar el remolque*—I have just cleaned the trailer
acabarse—to run out, to be out of; *se acabó el desinfectante*—we have run out of disinfectant
acariciar—to pet
accident—*el accidente*

accidente, el—accident
account—*la cuenta* (bill to be paid)
accountant—*el contador* (male),
  la contadora (female)
aceite, el—oil
aceite de hígado de bacalao, el—
  cod liver oil
acequia, la—irrigation ditch
ácido ascórbico, el—ascorbic acid
ácido graso, el—fatty acid
ácido láctico, el—lactic acid
add—*agregar, añadir*
additive—*el aditivo*
address—*la dirección*
aditivo, el—additive
administrar—to administrate
administrate—*administrar*
adónde—to where
adorable, cute—*precioso, preciosa*
after, afterward—*después*
afternoon—*la tarde*
again—*otra vez*
age—*la edad*
agent —*la agenta* (female),
  el agente (male)
agenta, la—agent (female)
agente, el—agent (male)
agosto—August
agregar—to add
agua, el—water
aguacero, el—thunderstorm;
  thundershower; downpour
ahora—now
ahora mismo—right now,
  immediately
ala, el or *la*—wing; *las alas*—
  wings
alambre, el—wire
alambre de púas, el—barbed wire
alfalfa—*la alfalfa*
alfalfa, la—alfalfa
alguien—someone
alimentación, la—food, feeding,

nourishment
alimentar—to feed, to nourish
alimentary tract—*el tracto
  alimenticio*
alimento, el—food, feed
alimento comercial, el—
  commercial feed
all, all of—*todo, toda*
allá—over there
allí—there, over there
almacén, el—barn, commodity
  barn
almacén de granos, el—grain
  elevator, grain storage
almidón, el— starch
almorzar (ue)—to eat lunch
almost—*casi*
almuerzo, el—lunch
already—*ya*
also—*también*
always—*siempre*
amable—kind, nice
amanecer—to wake up; literally,
  "to dawn"
ambiente controlado, el—
  controlled atmosphere
amiga, la—friend (female)
amigo, el—friend (male)
amilasa, la—amylase
amino acid—*el aminoácido*
aminoácido, el—amino acid
ampolla, la—blister
amylase—*la amilasa*
and—*y*
andar—to walk (humans);
  to run (machinery)
anemia—*la anemia*
anemia, la—anemia
anillo, el—leg band
animal—*el animal*
animal, el—animal
ano, el—anus; don't confuse
  this with *año*, which is "year"

anoche—last night
anochecer, el—nightfall
another—*otro, otra*
answer—*responder* (verb);
  la respuesta (noun)
anteayer—day before yesterday
antes—before; *que antes*—
  than before
antibacterial—*el bactericida*
antibiotic—*el antibiótico*
antibiótico, el—antibiotic
antioxidant—*el antioxidante*
antioxidante, el—antioxidant
anus—*el ano*
añadir—to add
añal, el—yearling
año, el—year; don't confuse this
  with *ano*, which is "anus"
apellido, el—last name
aplicador, el—applicator
aplicar—to apply
apple—*la manzana*
applicator—*el aplicador*
apply—*aplicar*
appointment—*la cita*
aprender—to learn
April—*abril*
apron—*el delantal*
aquel, aquella, aquello—
  way over there
aquí—here
área de monta, el—mating area
arenilla, la—grit, course sand
arete, el—ear tag
arete de la ala, el—wing tag,
  wing badge
arrive—*llegar*
arroyo, el—creek
artificial insemination—
  la inseminación artificial
as much—*tanto*
asa trompas, el—hog snare
ascorbic acid—*el ácido ascórbico*

ash—*la ceniza*
así—thus, like that
ask (for something)—*pedir (i, i)*
ask (a question)—*preguntar*
assail—*embestir*
at—*en*; (with time) *a*
atascar—to get stuck, to bog down
atropellar—to run over
auction—*el remate, la subasta*
August—*agosto*
aunt—*la tía*
auto, el—car, automobile
ave, el—fowl, bird; *las aves*—birds
avena, la—oats
aves de corral, las—poultry
avian cholera—*el cólera aviar*
aviario, el—aviary
aviary—*el aviario*
avicultura, la—poultry farming
awfully—*tremendo, tremenda*
ayer—yesterday
ayudar—to help
azadón, el—hoe
azúcar, el—sugar

B _____
baby—*el bebé, la bebita*
  (for humans)
back fat determination—*la
  determinación de la grasa dorsal*
bactericida, el—antibacterial
bad—*malo, mala*
badly—*mal*
balar—to bleat
balde, el—bucket
bale—*la paca*
baler—*la empacadora*
ballico, el—ryegrass
bandada, la—flock of birds
bandage—*vendar* (verb); *el
  vendaje* (noun)
bañar—to bathe, to dip
baño de inmersión, el—dipping bath

barbed wire—*el alambre de púas*
barley—*la cebada*
barn—*el almacén* (for grain);
  el establo (for animals)
barnyard—*el corral*
barrow—*el cerdo castrado*
báscula, la—scale; weighing crate
bathe—*bañar;* foot bath—
  el pediluvio; dipping bath—
  el baño de inmersión
be—*ser* or *estar* (see chapter 6)
bebé, el or *la bebita*—baby (humans)
bebedero, el—water trough; drinker
beber—to drink
becerrera, la—calf hutch; calf shed
becerro, el—calf (male);
  la becerra—calf (female)
bed—*la cama*
bedding—*la cama*
beef cattle—*el ganado de carne*
beet—*la remolacha*
before—*antes*
begin—*comenzar (ie), empezar (ie)*
believe—*creer*
Bermuda grass—*el pasto bermuda*
better—*mejor*
biberón, el—nipple bottle
bien—well; *usted maneja bien*—
  you drive well
bien hecho—well done
bienvenido, bienvenida—welcome
big—*grande*
bill—*la cuenta* (to be paid)
bin—*la caja*
bipartición de embriones, la—
  embryo splitting
bird—*el ave;* birds—*las aves*
birth—*el nacimiento* (humans);
  el parto (animals)
birth date—*la fecha de nacimiento*
bitácora, la—logbook
bite—*morder (ue)* (animals);
  picar (insects and snakes)

black—*negro, negra*
bladder—*la vesícula*
blanco, blanca—white
bleat—*balar*
blind—*ciego, ciega*
blister—*la ampolla*
block—*el bloque*
blood—*la sangre*
bloque, el—block
bluegrass—*el pasto azul*
boar—*el cerdo, el verraco*
board (a vehicle)—*subir*
bolo, el—bolus
bolo alimenticio, el—cud
bolus—*el bolo*
bomba, la—pump
bomba de gasolina, la—gas pump
bomba para lodos, la—manure
  pump
bonemeal—*la harina de huesos*
book—*el libro*
boots—*las botas*
boquilla, la—nozzle
boss—*el jefe* (male), *la jefa* (female)
botas, las—boots
botella, la—bottle
botiquín, el—first aid kit
bottle—*la botella;*
  nipple bottle—*el biberón*
bovine—*bovino, bovina*
bovino, bovina—bovine
box—*la caja* (cardboard)
box stall—*el cubículo*
boy—*el muchacho*
brake—*el freno*
bran—*el salvado*
brand—*marcar*
branding—*el marcaje*
branding iron—*el hierro de marcaje*
break—*romper*
breed—*la raza*
breeding system—*el sistema de*
  reproducción

brewer's yeast—*la levadura de cerveza*
bring—*traer*
broiler, broiling chicken—*el pollo de engorda*
broken—*roto, rota* (for animal bones); *descompuesto, descompuesta* (for machinery only)
bronchitis—*la bronquitis*
bronquitis, la—bronchitis
brooder—*la gallina clueca*
broom—*el cepillo*
brother—*el hermano*
brown—*pardo, parda*
Brown Swiss breed—*la raza pardo suiza*
brucellosis—*la brucelosis*
brucelosis, la—brucellosis
buche, el—crop, craw
buck (male goat)—*el macho cabrío* or *cabra macho, la*
bucket—*el balde, la cubeta*
buenas noches—good night
buenas tardes—good afternoon; note that afternoon extends to about seven or eight in the evening.
bueno, buena—good
buenos días—good morning
buey, el—ox
bull—*el toro*
buscar—to look for
but—*pero*
buy—*comprar*
buyer—*el comprador* (male), *la compradora* (female)

C _____

cabestro, el—halter
cabra, la—goat (female), doe
cabra hembra, la—female goat, doe
cabra macho, la—male goat, buck
cabrita, la—goat kid (female)
cabrito, el—goat kid (male)

cadena obstétrica, la—obstetric chain
caerse—to fall down
café, el—coffee; café
cage—*la jaula*
cage chute—*la trampa ajustable*
cage crate—*la trampa ajustable*
call—*llamar*
caja, la—bin; box
cajón, el—crate; dark box
cake—*la torta*
calcio, el—calcium
calcium—*el calcio*
calentador, el—heater
calentar—to heat
calf—*el ternero, la ternera; el becerro, la becerra*
calf hutch—*la becerrera*
calf shed—*la becerrera*
calidad, la—quality (importance); *alta calidad*—high quality
caliente—hot
call—*llamar; la llamada*
calm—*tranquilo, tranquila*
calor, el—heat
caloría, la—calorie
calorie—*la caloría*
cama, la—bed; bedding; straw litter
camada, la—litter (of newborn animals)
cambiar—to change
cambio, el—change
caminar—to walk
camino, el—road
camino de entrada, el—entrance road, driveway
camión, el—truck
camioneta, la—pickup truck
campo, el—countryside
can (able to, may)—*poder (ue)*
canastilla, la—canister
candle (eggs)—*mirar a trasluz*
canister—*la canastilla*

cansado, cansada—tired
caña, la—pipe; tube
capataz, el or *la*—foreman
capon—*el capón*
capón, el—capon
car—*el auto, el carro*
carbohidrato, el—carbohydrate
carbohydrate—*el carbohidrato*
care for—*cuidar de*
careful!—*¡cuidado!*
cargador, el—loader
cargar—to load
carnero, el—ram
carotene—*el caroteno*
caroteno, el—carotene
carretera, la—highway
carretilla, la—wheelbarrow
carrier—*el vehículo*
carro, el—car, automobile
carrot—*la zanahoria*
casa, la—house
casado, casada—married
cáscara, la—chaff; hull
casco, el—helmet, hoof
caseta, la—coop
casi—almost
cattle—*el ganado*
cattle ranch—*el rancho ganadero*
cattleman—*el ganadero*
cattle woman—*la ganadera*
caution—*el cuidado*
cazador, el—hunter
cebada, la—barley
cecum—*el ciego*
cellulose—*la celulosa*
celo, el—rut, in season; *está en celo*—it's in season, in rut
celulosa, la—cellulose
ceniza, la—ash
centeno, el—rye
cepillo, el—broom, push broom
cerca—near, close by
cerca, la—fence

cerca eléctrica, la—electrified fence
cerda, la—sow, female pig
cerda de reemplazo, la—gilt
cerdita, la—piglet (female)
cerdito, el—piglet (male)
cerdo, el—pig; boar
cerdo castrado, el—barrow
cerdo en crecimiento, el—growing swine
cerdo destetado, el—shoat, weaned piglet
cerdo en finalización, el—finishing swine
cereal—*el cereal*
cereal, el—cereal
cerradura, la—lock (the mechanism)
cerrar (ie)—to close
cerrar con llave—to lock up
cervix—*el cuello uterino*
chaff—*la cáscara*
change—*cambiar* (verb); *el cambio* (noun)
charca, la—pond
charge, assail—*embestir*
check—*el cheque* (bank check); to check over—*revisar*
cheque, el—check, bank check
chick—*el pollito* (male), *la pollita* (female)
chicken coop—*el gallinero*
chicken farm—*la granja avícola*
chico, chica—small (in size)
children—*los hijos* (sons, sons and daughters), *los niños* (children in general)
chiquero, el—pigsty
chiste, el—joke
cholera—*el cólera;* avian cholera—*el cólera aviar*
chop—*picar*
chopper—*la picadora*
chore—*el quehacer*

chute—*la manga, la rampa*
ciego, ciega—blind
ciego, el—cecum
ciencia, la—science
cita, la—appointment
citric pulp—*la pulpa de cítricos*
clavo, el—nail; *se tragó un*
    clavo—it swallowed a nail
clean—*limpiar* (verb); *limpio,*
    limpia (adjective)
client—*el* or *la cliente*
cliente, el or *la*—client
clima, el—climate, weather
climate—*el clima*
clip the needle teeth—*descolmillar*
cloaca—*la cloaca*
cloaca, la—cloaca
close—*cerrar (ie); cierre la*
    puerta—close the door
close by—*cerca*
cloudy—*nublado*
clover—*el trébol*
club—*el club*
club FFA, el—FFA (Future
    Farmers of America) Club
cobre, el—copper
cocinado, cocinada—cooked
cocinado, el—the cooked (food)
cod liver oil—*el aceite de hígado*
    de bacalao
coffee—*el café;* cup of coffee—
    una taza de café
cold—*frío, fría;* it's cold today—
    hace frío hoy
cojo, coja—lame; *la oveja está*
    coja—the ewe is lame
cólera, el—cholera
cólera aviar, el—avian cholera
colon—*el colon*
colon, el—colon
color—*el color*
color, el—color
collar—*el collar*

collar, el—collar; neck chain
combinada, la—combine
combinar—to combine
combine—*la combinada*
    (vehicle); *combinar* (verb)
come—*venir*
come back, return—*volver (ue)*
comedero, el—feed trough, feed
    bunk, feeder
comenzar (ie)—to begin
comer—to eat
comercial—commercial
commercial—*comercial*
commercial feed—*el alimento*
    comercial
commodity barn—*el almacén*
como—how; like, as; similar to
¿cómo?—how?; What did you say?
competición, la—tournament
comprador, el—buyer (male)
compradora, la—buyer (female)
comprar—to buy
comprender—*to understand*
computadora, la—computer
computer—*la computadora*
con—with
concentrado, el—concentrate
concentrate—*el concentrado*
coneja, la—rabbit (female)
conejito, el, conejita, la—baby rabbit
conejo, el—rabbit (male)
congratulations—*felicitaciones*
conocer—to know (a person);
    to know a fact is *saber*
consist of—*consistir en*
consistir en—to consist of
consume—*consumir*
consumir—to consume
consumo, el—consumption
consumption—*el consumo*
contador, el—accountant (male)
contadora, la—accountant (female)
contar (ue)—to count; to tell a story

contract—*el contrato*
contratación, la—hiring,
the act of hiring
contratar—to hire
contrato, el—contract
control—*el control*
control, el—control
controlled atmosphere—
el ambiente controlado
cooked—*cocinado, cocinada*
(adjective); *el cocinado* (noun)
coop—*la caseta;* chicken coop—
el gallinero
copper—*el cobre*
corazón, el—heart
corpus luteum—*el cuerpo lúteo*
cordera, la—lamb (female)
cordero, el—lamb (male)
corn—*el maíz*
corral—*el corral*
corral, el—corral; barnyard; pen
corral contenedor, el—holding pen
corral de engorda, el—feedlot
corral elevado, el—elevated stall
corral separador, el—sorting pen
corredor, el—passageway
correr—to run; when you're talking
about machinery rather than
humans or animals, use *andar*
cortapezuñas, el—sheep foot
trimmers
cortar—to cut
corto, corta—short (in length)
cosecha, la—harvest, crop
cosechadora, la—harvester
cosechar—to harvest
cost—*el costo, el precio* (noun);
costar (ue) (verb); *¿cuánto
cuesta?*—how much does it cost?
costar (ue)—to cost
costilla, la—rib
cottonseed cake—*la torta de
algodón*

cough—*toser*
count—*contar (ue)*
countryside—*el campo*
cousin—*el primo* (male),
la prima (female)
cover—*la cubierta* (noun);
cubrir (verb)
cow—*la vaca*
cowboy—*el vaquero*
cowgirl—*la vaquera*
cowman—*el vaquero*
cow woman—*la vaquera*
cowshed—*el establo*
coyote—*el coyote*
coyote, el—coyote
cracked—*quebrado, quebrada*
crate—*la jaula* (for animals)
craw—*el buche*
crazy—*loco, loca;* it drives me
crazy—*me vuelve loco*
creek—*el arroyo*
creer—to believe, to think
criovial, el—cryovial
crop—*la cosecha* (harvest);
el buche (in birds)
crude fat—*la grasa cruda*
crumbled—*en grano*
crushed—*triturado, triturada*
cryovial—*el criovial*
cualidad—quality (characteristic,
trait)
cuando—when
¿cuándo?—when?
¿cuánto? ¿cuánta?—how much?
how many?
cuarto—quarter hour; *es la una
y cuarto*—it's 1:15
cubeta, la—bucket
cubículo, el—box stall
cubierta, la—cover, lid
cubrir—to cover
cud—*el bolo alimenticio*
cuello uterino, el—cervix

cuenta, la—account, bill (to be paid)
cuero, el—leather; hide; pelt
cuerpo lúteo, el—corpus luteum
cuidado, el—care, caution;
¡*cuidado!*—watch out! careful!
cuidado del cordón umbilical,
    el—umbilical cord care
cuidar—to take care of, to watch
    out for
culebra, la—snake
cut—*cortar*
cute—*precioso, preciosa*
cyst—*el quiste*

D

dairy, dairy farm—*la granja lechera*
dairy cattle—*el ganado de leche*
danger—*el peligro*
dangerous—*peligroso, peligrosa*
dar—to give
dar de comer—to feed, nourish
dark box—*el cajón*
date—*la fecha*
daughter—*la hija*
day—*el día*
day before yesterday—*anteayer*
de—of; from; when *de* is next to
    el, they combine to form *del*
de nada—it's nothing, you're
    welcome (said after "thank you")
dead—*muerto, muerta*
debeak—*despicar*
debeaked—*despicado, despicada*
debeaking—*el despicado*
deber—to ought to
December—*diciembre*
decide—*decidir*
decidir—to decide
decir—to tell
dehorn—*descornar (ue)*
dehorned—*descornado, descornada*
dehorning—*el descornado*
dehulled—*descascarillado,*

descascarillada
dejar—to leave (behind)
delantal, el—apron
deliver—*entregar*
demasiado—too much
depend on—*depender de*
depender de—to depend on
desbarbillada—dewattled
desbarbillado, el—dewattling
desbarbillar—to dewattle
desbotonado, desbotonada—
    disbudded
desbotonado, el—disbudding
desbotonar—to disbud
descargar—to unload
descascarillado, descascarillada—
    dehulled
descolado, descolada—docktailed
descolado, el—tail docking
descolar—to dock the tail
descolmillado—clipping of the
    needle teeth
descolmillar—to clip the needle teeth
descompuesto, descompuesta—
    broken, broken down (for
    machinery only; otherwise,
    use *roto, rota* for "broken")
descornado, descornada—dehorned
descornado, el—dehorning
descornar (ue)—to dehorn
descremadora, la—separator (for milk)
descrestado, descrestada—dubbed
descrestado, el—dubbing
descrestar—to dub
desinfectante, el—disinfectant
desinfectar—to disinfect
despacio—slowly
despicado, el—debeaking
despicar—to debeak
desplumado, desplumada—plucked
desplumado, el—plucking
desplumar—to pluck
después—after, afterward

destetado, destetada—weaned
destetar—to wean
determinación de la grasa dorsal, la—back fat determination
devolver (ue)—to return (something loaned)
dewattle—*desbarbillar*
dewattled—*desbarbillado, desbarbillada*
dewattling—*el desbarbillado*
día, el—day
diarrea, la—diarrhea
diarrhea—*la diarrea*
diciembre—December
die—*morir (ue, u)*
diet—*la dieta*
dieta, la—diet
difficult—*difícil*
difficulty—*la dificultad*
difícil—difficult
dificultad, la—difficulty
digestive tract—*el tracto digestivo*
dipping bath—*el baño de inmersión*
dirección, la—address
disbud—*desbotonar*
disbudded—*desbotonado, desbotonada*
disbudding—*el desbotonado*
disinfect—*desinfectar*
disinfectant—*el desinfectante*
disparar—to shoot (a gun)
distribute—*repartir*
divorced—*divorciado, divorciada*
divorciado, divorciada—divorced
do—*hacer;* don't include in questions (see chapter 7 for the Spanish equivalent of "do" and "does" in questions)
docile—*manso, mansa*
dock the tail—*descolar*
docked tail—*descolado, descolada*
doctor—*el doctor* (male), *la doctora* (female)

doctor, *el*—doctor (male)
doctora, la—doctor (female)
doe (goat)—*la cabra, la cabra hembra;* (rabbit)—*la coneja*
dog—*el perro*
dólar, el—dollar
dollar—*el dólar*
domingo, el—Sunday
donde—where
¿dónde?—where?
door—*la puerta*
dormir (ue, u)—to sleep
dose—*la dosis*
dosis, la—dose
dot, on the dot—*en punto*
drink—*beber*
drinker—*el bebedero*
drive—*manejar* (a vehicle)
driver's license—*la licencia de manejo*
driveway—*el camino de entrada*
drop, droplet—*la gota*
droppings—*las heces*
dry—*seco, seca*
dry cow—*la vaca seca*
dry matter—*la materia seca*
dub—*descrestar*
dubbed—*descrestado, descrestada*
dubbing—*el descrestado*
duck—*el pato* (male), *la pata* (female)
duckling—*el patito* (male), *la patita* (female)
dueña, la—owner (female)
dueño, el—owner (male)
duodeno, el—duodenum
duodenum—*el duodeno*
duro, dura—hard

E _____

ear—*la oreja*
ear notching—*el muesqueo*
ear tag—*el arete*

early—*temprano*
east—*el este*
eat—*comer*
eat lunch—*almorzar (ue)*
eclosionar—to hatch
edad, la—age
egg—*el huevo*
electric clippers—*la esquiladora*
electrified fence—*la cerca eléctrica*
electrocutar—to electrocute
electrocute—*electrocutar*
electroejaculation—*la electroeyaculación*
electroeyaculación, la—electroejaculation
elevated stall—*el corral elevado*
emasculador, el—emasculator
emasculator—*el emasculador*
embestir—to assail, to charge
embrión, el—embryo
embrollado, embrollada—tangled
embrollar—to get tangled
embryo—*el embrión*
embryo sexing—*el sexado de embriones*
embryo splitting—*la bipartición de embriones*
embryo transfer—*la transferencia de embriones*
embudo, el—funnel
emergencia, la—emergency
emergency—*la emergencia*
empacadora, la—baler
empezar—begin
empujar—to push; *¡empuje!*—push!
en—in; on; at
en grano—crumbled
en punto—on the dot
encontrar (ue)—to meet; to run across
end—*terminar*
enero—January
enfermedad, la—illness, sickness
enfermo, enferma—ill, sick

English (language)—*el inglés*
enough—*suficiente* (quantity)
ensilado de sorgo, el—sorghum silage
ensilaje, el—silage
entender (ie)—to understand
entrada, la—entrance
entrance—*la entrada*
entregar—to deliver, to turn in, to hand over
enviar—to send
enzima, la—enzyme
enzyme—*la enzima*
epidemia, la—epidemic
epidemic—*la epidemia*
epidídimo, el—epididymis
epididymis—*el epidídimo*
equipment—*el equipo*
equipo, el—equipment
escape valve—*la válvula de escape*
escribir—to write
escroto, el—scrotum
escuela, la—school
ese, esa, eso—that (thing over there)
esófago, el—esophagus
esophagus—*el esófago*
español, el—Spanish language
esparcidora, la—spreader
esparcidora de estiércol, la—manure spreader
esparcir—to spread
esperar—to hope; to wait for
esperma, el—sperm
espermatozoide, el—spermatozoid
esposa, la—wife
esposo, el—husband
esquiladora, la—shearing clippers; electric clippers
esquilar—to shear
establo, el—stable; cowshed; animal barn
estabulado, estabulada—stabled
estabulado libre, el—free stall

168   *Dictionary*

estacionamiento, el—garage (for large vehicles)
estado civil, el—marital status
estar—to be (used with qualities that are changeable or are the result of an action)
este, el—east
este, esta, esto—this
estercolero, el—manure pile
esterilizado, esterilizada—sterilized
esterilizar—to sterilize
estiércol, el—manure
estómago, el—stomach
estro, el—estrus
estrogen—*el estrógeno*
estrógeno, el—estrogen
estropajo, el—mop
estrus—*el estro*
ewe—*la oveja, la oveja hembra*
examen, el—test
examinar—to examine
examine—*examinar*
exit—*la salida*
experience—*la experiencia*
experiencia, la—experience

F _____
fall down—*caerse*
faltar—to lack
familia, la—family
family—*la familia*
farm—*la finca, la granja*
farmacia, la—pharmacy
farrowing—*el parto*
farrowing crate—*la jaula de maternidad*
farrowing unit—*la maternidad*
fat—*la grasa* (noun); *gordo, gorda* (adjective)
father—*el padre*
fatty—(affectionate term) *gordito, gordita*

fatty acid—*el ácido graso*
faucet—*la llave*
feather—*la pluma*
febrero—February
February—*febrero*
feces—*las heces*
fecha, la—date; *la fecha de nacimiento*—birth date
fecundidad, la—fertility
feed—*alimentar, dar de comer* (verb); *el alimento* (noun)
feed bunk—*el comedero*
feeder—*el comedero*
feed trough—*el comedero*
feedlot—*el corral de engorda*
feeding—*la alimentación*
feedlot cattle—*el ganado estabulado*
feed mill—*el molino de alimento*
feel—*sentir (ie, i)*
felicitaciones—congratulations
female (animal)—*la hembra*
fence—*la cerca*
fence post—*el poste*
feo, fea—ugly
fértil—fertile
fertile—*fértil*
fertilidad, la—fertility
fertility—*la fertilidad, la fecundidad*
fertilización in vitro, la—in vitro fertilization
fertilizante, el—fertilizer
fertilizar—to fertilize
fertilize—*fertilizar*
fertilizer—*el fertilizante*
feto, el—fetus
fetus—*el feto*
fever—*la fiebre*
few—*poco, poca*
FFA (Future Farmers of America) Club—*el club FFA*
fiber—*la fibra*

fibra, la—fiber
fiebre, la—fever
fight—*pelear*
fill—*llenar*
filter—*el filtro*
filtro, el—filter
fin de semana, el—weekend
finally—*finalmente*
finalmente—finally
finca, la—farm
finish—*terminar*
finishing swine—*el cerdo en*
finalización
firma, la—signature
first aid—*los primeros auxilios*
first aid kit—*el botiquín*
first name—*el nombre de pila*
fistula—*la fístula*
fístula, la—fistula
flake—*la hojuela*
fleece, sheepskin—*el vellón*
flock—*la parvada* (of chickens);
la pavada (of turkeys);
la bandada (of birds);
el rebaño (of goats or sheep)
floor—*el suelo*
flour, meal—*la harina*
flu—*la influenza*
fodder—*el forraje, el pienso*
fodder crops—*las plantas forrajeras*
fogoso, fogosa—spirited, frisky
fold, sheepfold—*el redil*
follicle-stimulating hormone—
la hormona folículo-estimulante
or *la hormona estimulante del*
folículo
follow—*seguir (i, i)*
food—*el alimento, la alimentación*
foot—*la pata* (animals); *el pie*
(humans)
foot bath—*el pediluvio*
for—*para*
foreman—*el* or *la capataz; el* or
la mayordomo

fork, pitchfork—*la horquilla,*
el trinchete
forklift—*el montacargas*
forage—*el forraje*
forraje, el—forrage, fodder
fósforo, el—phosphorus
foto período, el—photo period
fowl—*el ave*
fracturar—to fracture
fracture—*fracturar*
frecuentemente—frequently
free stall—*el estabulado libre*
freno, el—rope halter; brake
frequently—*frecuentemente*
Friday—*el viernes*
friend—*el amigo* (male),
la amiga (female)
frío, el—cold; *hace frío*—it's cold
frío, fría—cold (used with estar)
frisky—*fogoso, fogosa*
from—*de;* when *de* is next to *el,*
they combine to form *del*
full—*lleno, llena*
función, la—function
funcionar—to function
function—*funcionar* (verb);
la función (noun)
fungicida, el—fungicide
fungicide—*el fungicida*
funnel—*el embudo*

G _____

gallbladder—*la vesícula biliar*
gallina, la—hen
gallina clueca, la—brooder
gallina de postura, la—layer,
laying hen
gallinero, el—henhouse, chicken coop
gallo, el—rooster
game (of sports)—*el partido*
ganadera, la—cattlewoman
ganadero, el—cattleman
ganado, el—cattle, herd

ganado de carne, el—beef cattle
ganado de leche, el—dairy cattle
ganado en pastoreo, el—grazing cattle
ganado estabulado, el—feedlot cattle
gano do porcino, el—swine herd
garage—*el garaje; el estacionamiento*
   (for large vehicles)
garaje, el—garage
garden—*el jardín*
garrapata, la—tick
gas pump—*la bomba de gasolina*
gasolina, la—gasoline
gasoline—*la gasolina*
gastric juice—*el jugo gástrico*
gate—*la puerta*
generally—*generalmente*
generalmente—generally
germ—*el germen*
germen, el—germ
gestación, la—gestation
gestation—*la gestación*
gilt—*la cerda de reemplazo*
girl—*la muchacha*
give—*dar*
give birth—*parir*
give food—*dar de comer*
gizzard—*la molleja*
gland—*la glándula*
glándula, la—gland
glándula mamaria, la—
   mammary gland
glasses (eye)—*los lentes;*
   protective glasses, safety
   glasses—*los lentes protectores*
gloves—*los guantes*
gluten, el—glutin
glutin—*el gluten*
go—*ir;* go for (fetch or bring
   back)—*recogar;* go up—*subir*
goat—*la cabra; el macho cabrío*
   or *la cabra macho* (male);
   la cabra, la cabra hembra
   (female)

goat, kid—*el cabrito, la cabrita*
going to (do something)—*ir a +*
   infinitive
gonadotropina sérica de la yegua
   preñada, la—pregnant mare
   serum gonadotropin
good—*bueno, buena*
good afternoon—*buenas tardes*
good morning—*buenos días*
good night—*buenas noches*
gordito, gordita—fat, fatty
   (affectionate term)
gordo, gorda—fat
gota, la—droplet, drop
gracias—thank you
gracias a dios—thank god
grain—*el grano*
grain bin—*el granero*
grain elevator—*el almacén de*
   granos, el silo con elevador
grain storage—*el granero*
grains—*en grano*
granary—*el granero*
granddaughter—*la nieta*
grande—big; grown up
   (for humans only)
grandson—*el nieto*
granero, el—granary; barn;
   grain bin
granja, la—farm
granja avícola, la—chicken farm
granja lechera, la—dairy farm
granja porcícola, la—hog farm
grano, el—grain, seed; grain, particle
grasa, la—fat
grasa cruda, la—crude fat
grasa dorsal, la—back fat
grass—*la hierba, el pasto*
grasshopper—*el saltamontes*
grave—serious, grave; close to death
grazing—*el pastoreo*
grazing cattle—*el ganado en pastoreo*
greetings—*los saludos*

grind—*moler (ue)*
grit—*la arenilla*
grits—*la sémola*
ground, ground up—*molido, molida*
growing swine—*el cerdo en crecimiento*
growing-finishing unit—*la unidad de crecimiento-finalización*
grown up—*grande*
guajolote, el—turkey (in Mexico)
guantes, los—gloves
gustar—to please; *me gusta*—I like it (literally, "it pleases me").

H _____

haber—to have (done something); used with the before-now verbs
hablar—to speak
hacer—to do; to make
half—*la mitad; media*
hallway—*el pasillo*
halter—*el cabestro*
hambre, el—hunger; *tengo hambre*—I'm hungry
hand—*la mano* (for humans); *la pata* (for animals)
happen—*pasar, ocurrir, suceder*
hard—*duro, dura*
harina, la—flour; meal (such as bonemeal)
harina de huesos, la—bonemeal
harvest—*la cosecha* (noun); *cosechar* (verb)
harvester—*la cosechadora*
hasta—until
hatch—*eclosionar*
hato, el—herd (cattle)
have—*tener* (to own); *haber* (used with before-now verbs)
have just—*acabar de*
have to—*tener que*
hay—there is, there are
hay—*el heno*

hay swather—*la segadora*
hayloft—*el henil*
haystack—*el pajar*
health—*la salud*
hear—*oír;* did you hear that?—*¿sintió eso?*
heart—*el corazón*
heat—*calentar* (verb); *el calor* (noun)
heat patch—*el parche detector de calores*
heater—*el calentador*
heces, las—feces, droppings
heifer—*la vaquilla, la novilla*
helmet—*el casco*
help—*ayudar*
help!—*¡socorro!*
hembra, la—female of the species
hen—*la gallina*
henhouse—*el gallinero*
henil, el—hayloft
heno, el—hay
herd—(noun) *el ganado, el hato* (cattle); *el rebaño* (goats or sheep); *la piara* (pigs)
herd—(verb) *reunir*
herder—*el pastor* (male), *la pastora* (female)
here—*aquí, acá*
herida, la—wound, injury
hermana, la—sister
hermano, el—brother
hide—*la piel, el cuero*
hierba, la—grass
hierba callera, la—sedum
hierro, el—iron
hierro a marcar, el—branding iron
hígado, el—liver
highway—*la carretera*
hija, la—daughter
hijo, el—son
hilo, el—wire
hire—*contratar*

hiring—*la contratación*
(the act of hiring)
hocico, el—muzzle
hoe—*el azadón*
hog—*el porcino*
hog farm—*la granja porcícola*
hog snare—*el asa trompas*
hojuela, la—flake
holding pen—*el corral contenador*
hole in the ground—*el hoyo*
hombre, el—man
hoof—*la pezuña, el casco*
hope—*esperar*
hora, la—hour
hormona, la—hormone
hormona estimulante del folículo, la—
follicle-stimulating hormone
hormona folículo-estimulante, la—
follicle-stimulating hormone
hormona luteinizante, la—
luteinizing hormone
hormone—*la hormona*
horquilla, la—fork, pitchfork
hose, water hose—*la manguera*
hospital—*el hospital*
hospital, el—hospital
hot—*caliente;* it's a hot day—
hace calor
hour—*la hora*
house—*la casa*
how—*como;* how?—*¿cómo?*
how much?—*¿cuánto?;* how
many?—*¿cuánto? ¿cuánta?*
hoy—today
hoyo, el—hole in the ground
huerta, la—orchard (large)
huerto, el—orchard (small,
family-size)
huevo, el—egg
hull—*la cáscara;* dehulled—
descascarillado, descascarillada
hunger—*el hambre;*
I'm hungry—*Tengo hambre*

hunter—*el cazador*
husband—*el marido, el esposo*

I _____

idioma, el—language
íleo, el—ileum
ileum—*el íleo*
ill—*enfermo, enferma*
illness—*la enfermedad*
important—*importante*
importante—important
improve—*mejorar*
in—*en*
in vitro fertilization—
la fertilización in vitro
incubadora, la—incubator
incubator—*la incubadora*
industria, la—industry
industria avícola, la—poultry
industry
industria porcina, la—swine
industry
industry—*la industria*
infect—*infectar*
infectar—to infect
infertilidad, la—infertility
infertility—*la infertilidad*
informe, el—report
influenza, la—flu
infundíbulo, el—infundibulum
infundibulum—*el infundíbulo*
ingerido, ingerida—ingested
ingerir—to ingest
ingest—*ingerir*
ingested—*ingerido, ingerida*
inglés, el—English language
ingredient—*el ingrediente*
ingrediente, el—ingredient
injection—*la inyección*
injury—*la herida*
inseminación artificial, la—
artificial insemination
inseminar—to inseminate

inseminate—*inseminar*
inspeccionar—to inspect
inspect—*inspeccionar*
inspector—*el inspector* (male),
   la inspectora (female)
inspector, el—inspector (male)
inspectora, la—inspector (female)
instalaciones de esquilar, las—
   shearing facilities
instrucciones, las—instructions
instruction book—*el manual*
instructions—*las instrucciones*
insurance—*el seguro*
intestino delgado, el—small intestine
intestino grueso, el—large intestine
inyección, la—injection, shot
inyección de hierro, la—iron shot
iodine—*el yodo*
ir—to go; *ir a* + infinitive—
   going to (do something)
iron—*el hierro*
iron shot—*la inyección de hierro*
irrigation ditch—*la acequia*

J
jabón (often spelled *javón*), *el*—soap
jalar—to pull (Mexico);
   ¡jale!—pull!
January—*enero*
jardín, el—garden
jaula, la—cage, crate
jaula de maternidad, la—
   farrowing crate
jaula de postura, la—laying cage
jefa, la—boss (female)
jefe, el—boss (male)
jejunum—*el yeyuno*
job—*el puesto, el trabajo*
joke—*el chiste;* to tell a joke—
   decir un chiste or *contar un chiste*
jueves, el—Thursday
jugar (ue)—to play
jugo gástrico, el—gastric juice

julio—July
July—*julio*
June—*junio*
junio—June

K
keep going—*seguir (i, i)*
key—*la llave*
kid—*el cabrito* (male goat), *la cabrita*
   (female goat); *el niño* (male child),
   la niña (female child)
kind, nice—*amable*
know—*conocer* (a person); *saber*
   (a fact, how to do something)

L
lack—*faltar*
lactación, la—lactation
lactasa, la—lactase
lactase—*la lactasa*
lactation—*la lactación*
lactic acid—*el ácido láctico*
lamb—*el cordero* (male),
   la cordera (female)
lame—*cojo, coja*
lana, la—wool
lane; runway—*la línea, el pasillo*
language—*el idioma*
large intestine—*el intestino grueso*
largo, larga—long
lasso—*el lazo*
last name—*el apellido*
last night—*anoche*
last week—*la semana pasada*
late—*tarde*
lately—*últimamente*
later—*más tarde*
lavar—to wash
lay (eggs)—*poner*
layer, laying hen—*la gallina de*
   postura
layer parent stock—*el reproductor*
   de postura

laying cage—*la jaula de postura*
lazo, el—lasso
learn—*aprender*
leather—*el cuero*
leave (go out)—*salir*
leave (behind)—*dejar*
leche, la—milk
lechería, la—building for
    processing or selling milk
lechón, el—piglet; shoat (male)
lechona, la—piglet; shoat (female)
leer—to read
leg—*la pierna*
leg band—*el anillo*
lentes, los—glasses (eye)
lentes protectores, los—
    protective glasses
lesion—*la lesión*
lesión, la—lesion
less—*menos*
levadura de cerveza, la—brewer's
    yeast
libro, el—book
licencia de manejo, la—
    driver's license
lid—*la cubierta*
life—*la vida*
lightning—*el relámpago*
lignin—*la lignina*
lignina, la—lignin
like—*gustar* (literally, "to please");
    I like it—*me gusta*
like, as—*como*
limpiar—to clean
limpio, limpia—clean
lindo, linda—pretty; handsome;
    beautiful
línea, la—runway; lane
lípidos, los—lipids
lipids—*los lípidos*
liquid nitrogen tank—*el tanque
    de nitrógeno líquido*
listo, lista—ready, prepared

liter—*el litro*
litro, el—liter
litter—*la camada* (newborn animals);
    la cama (straw litter)
little—*pequeño, pequeña; chico,
    chica*; a little—*un poco*
live—*vivir*
liver—*el hígado*
llamar—to call
llamarse—to call oneself, to be named
llanta, la—tire (on a vehicle)
llave, la—key; wrench; faucet
llegar—to arrive
llenar—to fill
lleno, llena—full
llover (ue)—to rain
lluvia, la—rain
lo siento—I'm sorry
load—*cargar;* unload—*descargar*
loader—*el cargador, el montacargas*
loading chute—*la rampa de
    embarque, la manga de
    embarque*
loading ramp—*la rampa de carga*
loan—*prestar*
local de ordeño, el—milking shed
lock—*la cerradura*
lock up—*cerrar (ie) con llave*
lockup; cage crate; cage chute—
    la trampa ajustable
loco, loca—crazy, nuts; *me vuelve
    loco*—it drives me nuts
lodo, el—mud
logbook—*la bitácora*
look—*mirar;* look like, seem—
    parecer
look over, check over—*revisar*
long—*largo, larga*
look for—*buscar*
lose—*perder (ie)*
a lot—*mucho*
lunch—*el almuerzo;* to eat
    lunch—*almorzar (ue)*

lunes, el—Monday
luteinizing hormone—
  la hormona luteinizante

M _____
machine—*la máquina*
machinery—*la maquinaria,*
  el equipo
macho, el—male animal
macho cabrío, el—male goat, buck
magnesio, el—magnesium
magnesium—*el magnesio*
maíz, el—corn
make—*hacer*
mal—badly
male animal—*el macho*
malo, mala—bad
mamá, la—mother, mom (the
  more formal *madre* isn't used
  much in conversation)
mammary gland—*la glándula*
  mamaria
man—*el hombre*
¿mande?—what did you say?
  (Mexico)
manejar—to drive (a vehicle)
manga, la—chute; literally, "sleeve"
manga de embarque—loading chute
manga separadora, la—sorting chute
manganese—*el manganeso*
manganeso, el—manganese
manguera, la—hose; water hose
mano, la—hand (for humans;
  la pata for animals)
manso, mansa—docile, tame
manual, instruction book—
  el manual
manual, el—manual, instruction book
manure—*el estiércol*
manure pile—*el estercolero*
manure pump—*la bomba para lodos*
manure separator—*el separador*
  de estiércol

manure spreader—*la esparcidora*
  de estiércol
many—*mucho, mucha*
manzana, la—apple
mañana—tomorrow
mañana, la—morning
máquina, la—machine
maquinaria, la—machinery
marcaje, el—branding
marcar—to brand
March—*marzo*
mare—*la yegua*
marido, el—husband
marital status—*el estado civil*
married—*casado, casada*
martes, el—Tuesday
marzo—March
más—more; *más tarde*—later
máscara, la—mask
mash (feed)—*el puré*
mask—*la máscara*
mastitis—*la mastitis*
mastitis, la—mastitis
materia seca, la—dry matter
maternidad, la—farrowing unit
mating area—*el área de monta*
maybe—*quizás*
mayordomo, el or *la*—foreman
meal—*la harina;* bonemeal—
  la harina de huesos
measure—*medir (i, i)*
media, la—half; *son las tres y*
  media—it's 3:30 (literally,
  "three and a half hours")
medianoche, la—midnight
médica, la—physician (female)
medicina, la—medicine
medicine—*la medicina*
médico, el—physician (male)
medio—partly; *medio nublado*—
  partly cloudy
mediodía, el—noon
medir (i, i)—to measure

meet—*encontrar (ue)*
mejor—better
mejorar—to improve
melaza, la—molasses
member (of a club)—*el socio*
    (male), *la socia* (female)
menos—less; minus
mes, el—month
mesa, la—table
metano, el—methane
methane—*el metano*
mezcla, la—mix
mezcladora, la—mixer
mezclar—to mix
Mexican—*mexicano, mexicana*
mexicano, mexicana—Mexican
midnight—*la medianoche*
miércoles, el—Wednesday
mijo, el—millet
milk—*la leche* (noun);
    ordeñar (verb)
milk cow—*la vaca lechera*
milk-processing or -selling
    building—*la lechería*
milker—*el ordeñador* (male),
    la ordeñadora (female)
milking—*el ordeño*
milking machine—*la ordeñadora*
milking parlor—*la sala de ordeño*
milking shed—*el local de ordeño*
Milking Shorthorn breed—*la
    raza cuernos cortos lechera*
milking system—*el sistema de ordeño*
millet—*el mijo, el millo*
millo, el—millet
mineral—*el mineral*
mineral, el—mineral
minus—*menos*
mirar—to watch, to look
mirar a trasluz—to candle
mismo, misma—same
mitad, la—half (such as half of a pie)
mix—*la mezcla* (noun); *mezclar* (verb)

mixer—*la mezcladora*
molasses—*la melaza*
moler (ue)—to grind
molido, molida—ground, ground up
molino de alimento, el—feed mill
molleja, la—gizzard
moment—*el momento*
momento, el—moment
Monday—*el lunes*
monogastric—*el monogástrico*
monogástrico, el—monogastric
montacargas, el—forklift; loader
montar—to mount
month—*el mes*
moo—*mugir*
mop—*el estropajo*
morder (ue)—to bite
more—*más*
morir (ue, u)—to die
morning—*la mañana*
mostrar (ue)—to show
mother, mom—*la mamá*
mount—*montar*
move—*mover (ue)*
mover (ue)—to move
much—*mucho;* as much, that
    much—*tanto*
muchacha, la—girl
muchacho, el—boy
mucho—a lot, much
mucho, mucha—many
mucho gusto—pleased to meet you
mud—*el lodo*
muda, la—shearing shed
muerto, muerta—dead
muesqueo, el—ear notching
mugir—to moo
multitud, la—multitude
multitude—*la multitud*
muy—very
muy amable—how kind of you
muy bien—very well
muzzle—*el hocico*

N
nacimiento, el—birth (humans);
   el parto (animals)
nada—nothing
nail—*la uña* (toenail); *el clavo*
   (for hammering)
nariguero, el—nose tongs
navaja, la—pocket knife
navel—*el ombligo*
near, nearby—*cerca*
necesario, necesaria—necessary
necesitar—to need
necessary—*necesario, necesaria*
need—*necesitar*
negro, negra—black
neck chain—*el collar*
neighbor—*el vecino* (male),
   la vecina (female)
nephew—*el sobrino*
nest—*el nido*
nevar (ie)—to snow
never—*nunca*
new—*nuevo, nueva*
newborn—*recién nacido, recién*
   nacida
news—*las noticias*
niacin—*la niacina*
niacina, la—niacin
nice—*simpático, simpática*
   (humans only)
nido, el—nest
niece—*la sobrina*
nieta, la—granddaughter
nieto, el—grandson
night—*la noche*
nightfall—*el anochecer*
niña, la—girl; *niño, el*—boy;
   niños, los—children
nipple bottle—*el biberón*
no hay de qué—you're welcome,
   it's nothing (said in reply to
   "thank you")
noche, la—night

nombre de pila, el—first name
noon—*el mediodía*
nopal, el—prickly pear cactus
   (in Mexico)
normal—*normal*
norte, el—north
north—*el norte*
nose tongs—*el nariguero*
nostril—*el ollar*
nothing—*nada;* it's nothing—
   de nada, no hay de qué
noticias, las—news
nourish—*alimentar, dar de comer*
nourishment—*la alimentación*
November—*noviembre*
noviembre—November
novilla, la—heifer
novillo, el—steer
now—*ahora;* right now—*ahora*
   mismo
nozzle—*la boquilla*
nublado, nublada—cloudy
nuevo, nueva—new
number—*el número*
número, el—number
nunca—never
nutrient—*el nutriente*
nutriente, el—nutrient
nutrióloga, la—nutritionist
   (female)
nutriólogo, el—nutritionist (male)
nutritional value—*el valor nutritivo*
nutritionist—*el nutriólogo* (male),
   la nutrióloga (female)

O
o—or
oats—*la avena*
obesidad, la—obesity
obesity—*la obesidad*
obrera, la—worker (female)
obrero, el—worker (male)
obstetric chain—*la cadena obstétrica*

occur—*ocurrir, pasar, suceder*
October—*octubre*
octubre—October
ocurrir—ocurr
oeste, el—west
of—*de;* when *de* is next to *el,*
    they combine to form *del*
often—*a menudo*
oil—*el aceite*
oil cake—*la torta oleaginosa*
ointment—*el ungüento*
oír—to hear
old—*viejo, vieja*
ollar, el—nostril
omaso, el—omasum
omasum—*el omaso*
ombligo, el—navel
on—*en*
only, one and only—*único, única*
oocyte—*el ovocito*
open—*abrir* (verb); *abierto, abierta*
    (adjectives; use with *estar: la puerta
    está abierta*—the gate is open)
or—*o*
orchard—*la huerta* (large),
    el huerto (small)
ordeñador, el—milker (male)
ordeñadora, la—milker (female);
    milking machine
ordeñar—to milk
ordeño, el—milking
oreja, la—ear
organización, la—organization
organizar—to organize
organization—*la organización*
organize—*organizar*
other—*otro, otra*
otra vez—again
otro, otra—other, another
ought—*deber*
ovario, el—ovary
ovary—*el ovario*
oveja, la—sheep

oveja hembra, la—ewe
over there—*allá, allí*
overalls—*el overol*
overol, el—overalls
oviduct—*el oviducto*
oviducto, el—oviduct
ovocito, el—oocyte
ovulación, la—ovulation
ovulation—*la ovulación*
owner—*el dueño* (male),
    la dueña (female)
ox—*el buey*
oxitocina, la—oxytocin
oxytocin—*la oxitocina*

P _____

paca, la—bale
padre, el—father
padres, los—parents
pagar—to pay
paja, la—straw
pajar, el—haystack
pajilla, la—straw (used in
    reproduction)
pala, la—shovel
palpación, la—palpation
palpation—*la palpación*
pancreas—*el páncreas*
páncreas, el—pancreas
papel, el—paper
paper—*el papel*
para—in order to, so that; for
parche detector de calores, el—
    heat patch
pardo, parda—brown
pardon—*perdonar;* pardon me—
    perdóneme
parecer—to seem; to look like
parents—*los padres*
pariente, el or la—relative,
    member of the family
parir—to give birth
partido, el—game of sports

partly—*medio*
partly cloudy—*medio nublado*
parto, el—birth, farrowing,
  parturition
parturition—*el parto*
parvada, la—flock of chickens
pasado, pasada—past;
  la semana pasada—last week
pasar—to happen, to occur
pasillo, el—passageway, hallway;
  lane; runway
past—*pasado, pasada*
pasterizadora, la—pasteurizer
pasteurizer—*la pasterizadora*
pastizal, el—pasture, grazing land
passageway—*el pasillo, el corredor*
pasto, el—grass; pasture
pasto azul, el—bluegrass
pasto bermuda, el—Bermuda grass
pasto Sudán, el—Sudan grass
pastor, el—herder, shepherd (male)
pastora, la—herder, shepherd
  (female)
pastoreo, el—grazing
pastura, la—pasture
pasture—*el pastizal, el pasto,*
  la pastura
pata, la—paw, foot (used for
  animals); duck (female)
patita, la—duckling (female)
patito, el—duckling (male)
pato, el—duck (male)
pava, la—turkey hen
pavada, la—flock of turkeys
pavo, el—turkey tom
paw—*la pata*
pay—*pagar*
pediluvio, el—footbath
pedir (i, i)—to ask for, to ask a favor;
  to ask a question is *preguntar*
pelear—to fight
pelets, los—pellets
peligro, el—danger

peligroso, peligrosa—dangerous
pellets—*los pelets*
pelt—*la piel, el cuero*
pene, el—penis
penis—*el pene*
pensar (ie)—to think
peor—worse
pequeño, pequeña—small (in size)
per—*por*
perch—*la percha*
percha, la—perch
perder (ie)—to lose
perdonar—to pardon, to forgive;
  perdóneme—pardon me
pero—but
perro, el—dog
pesar—to weigh
pesebre, el—stall
peso, el—weight
pesticida, el—pesticide
pesticide—*el pesticida*
pet—*acariciar* (verb)
pezón, el—teat
pezonera, la—teat cup
pezuña, la—hoof
pharmacy—*la farmacia*
phosphorus—*el fósforo*
photo period—*el foto período*
physician—*el médico* (male),
  la médica (female)
piara, la—herd of pigs
picadora, la—chopper
picar—to chop; to bite, to sting
  (snakes and insects)
pick up—*recoger;* he went to pick
  up the mail—*fue para recoger*
  el correo
pickup truck—*la camioneta;*
  la troca (U.S. slang)
pie, el—foot (in humans)
piel, la—skin, hide
pienso, el—fodder
pierna, la—leg

pig—*el cerdo* (male); also *el verraco* (often spelled *berraco*); *la cerda, la vientre* (female)
piglet—*el lechón, la lechona; el cerdito, la cerdita*
pigsty—*la pocilga, el chiquero*
pipe—*la caña* (plumbing); *el tubo*
pitchfork—*la horquilla, el trinchete*
plantas forrajeras, las—fodder crops
play—*jugar (ue)* (games, sports); *tocar* (music)
please—*por favor*
please—*gustar;* I like it (literally, "it pleases me")—*me gusta*
pleased to meet you—*mucho gusto*
pluck—*desplumar*
plucked—*desplumado, desplumada*
plucking—*el desplumado*
pluma, la—feather
plumage—*el plumaje*
plumaje, el—plumage
pocilga, la—pigsty
pocket knife—*la navaja*
poco, poca—few; *un poco*—a little
poder (ue)—to be able
poligástrico—polygastric
polla, la—pullet (female)
polla de reemplazo, la—replacement pullet
pollera, la—poultry dealer (female)
pollero, el—poultry dealer (male)
pollita, la—chick (female)
pollito, el—chick (male)
pollo, el—pullet (male)
pollo de engorda, el—broiler, broiling chicken
pollo para asar, el—roaster, roasting chicken
polygastric—*poligástrico*
pond—*la charca*
poner—to put; to lay (eggs)
ponerse—to put on (clothes)

por—per
por favor—please
porcino, el—hog
pork—*el puerco*
posible—possible
position (job)—*el puesto*
possible—*posible;* it's possible—*es posible*
poste, el—fence post
potasio, el—potassium
potassium—*el potasio*
poultry—*las aves de corral*
poultry dealer—*el pollero* (male), *la pollera* (female)
poultry farming—*la avicultura*
poultry industry—*la industria avícola*
pozo, el—water well
precio, el—price, cost
precioso, preciosa—adorable, cute
prefer—*preferir (ie, i)*
preferir (ie, i)—to prefer
pregnant—*preñada* (in animals only); *está preñada*—it's pregnant; for humans, use *embarazada*
pregnant mare serum gonadotropin —*la gonadotropina sérica de la yegua preñada*
preguntar—to ask a question; to ask for something use *pedir*
premezcla, la—premix
premix—*la premezcla*
prensa, la—squeeze chute
preñada—pregnant (in animals only)
preparar—to prepare
prepare—*preparar*
prepared—*preparado, preparada,* or *listo, lista*
prestar—to loan
pretty—*lindo, linda*
price—*el precio*

prickly pear cactus—*el nopal*
(in Mexico), *la tuna*
prima, la—cousin (female)
primeros auxilios, los—first aid
primo, el—cousin (male)
problem—*el problema*
problema, el—problem
producción, la—production
produce—*producir, rendir (i, i)*
producir—to produce
production—*la producción*
productive—*productivo, productiva*
productivo, productiva—productive
progesterona, la—progesterone
progesterone—*la progesterona*
program—*el programa*
programa, el—program
*programa libre de patógenos
específicos, el*—Specific
Pathogen-Free (SPF) Program
progresar—to progress
progress—*progresar*
prometer—to promise
promise—*prometer*
pronto—soon
prostaglandin—*la prostaglandina*
prostaglandina, la—prostaglandin
próstata, la—prostate
prostate—*la próstata*
protect—*proteger;* to protect
oneself—*protegerse*
protective—*protector, protectora*
protective glasses—*los lentes
protectores*
protector, protectora—protective
proteger—to protect
protegerse—to protect oneself
protein—*la proteína*
proteína, la—protein
prueba, la—test
puerco, el—pork
puerta, la—door, gate
puesto, el—job, position

pull—*jalar* (Mexico); pull!—*¡jale!*
pullet—*el pollo* (male), *la polla*
(female)
pulpa de cítricos, la—citric pulp
pump—*la bomba*
puré, el—mash, mashed food
pus—*el pus;* in Mexico, *la pus*
pus, el—pus; in Mexico, *la pus*
push—*empujar;* push!—*¡empuje!*
push broom—*el cepillo*
put—*poner*
put on (clothes)—*ponerse*

Q

quality—*la cualidad* (characteristic,
trait); *la calidad* (importance);
high quality—*alta calidad*
quarter hour—*cuarto;* it's 1:15—
es la una y cuarto
que—that, which
¿qué?—what?
quebrado, quebrada—cracked
quehacer, el—task, chore
querer (ie)—to want
quien—who
¿quién?—who?
quiste, el—cyst
quizás—maybe

R

rabbit—*el conejo* (male),
la coneja (female), *el conejito,
la conejita* (baby rabbit)
ración, la—ration
rain—*llover (ue)* (verb); *la lluvia*
(noun)
rake—*el rastrillo*
ram—*el carnero*
ramp—*la rampa*
rampa, la—ramp, chute
rampa de carga—loading ramp
rampa de embarque—loading chute
ranch—*el rancho*

ranch owner—*el ranchero,
la ranchera*
ranchera, la—ranch owner (female)
ranchero, el—ranch owner (male)
rancho, el—ranch
rancho ganadero, el—cattle ranch
rancho ovejero, el—sheep ranch
rancid—*rancio, rancia*
rancio, rancia—rancid
raspado, raspada—scratched
raspador, el—scraper
rastrillo, el—rake
rastrojo, el—stubble
ration—*la ración*
raza, la—breed
raza cuernos cortos lechera, la—
Milking Shorthorn breed
raza pardo suiza, la—Brown
Swiss breed
read—*leer*
ready—*listo, lista*
rebaño, el—flock (of sheep or goats)
receipt—*el recibo*
receive—*recibir*
recently—*últimamente*
recibir—to receive
recibo, el—receipt
recién nacido, recién nacida—
newborn
recoger—to pick up; to go for; to
gather; *fue a recoger el correo*—
he went to pick up the mail
recomendar (ie)—to recommend
recommend—*recomendar (ie)*
recto, el—rectum
rectum—*el recto*
red—*rojo, roja*
redil, el—sheep pen; fold
register—*registrar*
registrar—to register
relámpago, el—lightning
relative, member of the family—
el or *la pariente*

remate, el—auction
remolacha, la—beet
remolque, el—trailer
render—*rendir (i, i)*
rendir (i, i)—to yield, to render,
to produce
repair—*reparar*
reparar—to repair
repartir—to distribute
repeat—*repetir (i, i)*
repetir (i, i)—to repeat
replacement pullet—*la polla de
reemplazo*
report—*el informe*
representante, el or *la*—
representative
representative—*el* or *la
representante*
reproducción, la—reproduction
reproduction—*la reproducción*
reproductor de postura, el—
layer parent stock
resist—*resistir*
resistir—to resist
respond—*responder*
responder—to respond, to answer
resultados, los—results
results—*los resultados*
retículo, el—reticulum
reticulum—*el retículo*
return—*volver (ue)* (to come
back); *devolver (ue)*—to
return (something loaned)
reunir—to herd; to gather up
revisar—to check over; to look over
revolcadero, el—wallow
rib—*la costilla*
riboflavin—*la riboflavina*
riboflavina, la—riboflavin
right now—*ahora mismo*
río, el—river
river—*el río*
road—*el camino*

roaster, roasting chicken—*el pollo para asar*
rociador, el—sprayer
rociar—to spray
rojo, roja—red
rolado, rolada—rolled
rolled—*rolado, rolada*
romper—to break
rooster—*el gallo*
rope—*la soga*
rope halter—*el freno*
roto, rota—broken (animal bones)
rumen—*el rumen*
rumen, el—rumen
rumia, la—rumination
rumiante, el—ruminant
rumiar—to ruminate
ruminant—*el rumiante*
ruminate—*rumiar*
rumination—*la rumia*
run—*correr* (humans and animals); *andar* (machinery)
run across (someone)—*encontrar (ue)*
run out—*acabarse*
run over (with a vehicle)—*atropellar*
runway, lane—*la línea, el pasillo*
rut—*el celo;* in rut—*en celo*
rye—*el centeno*
ryegrass—*el ballico,* "ryegrass"

S

sábado, el—Saturday
saber—to know (a fact); to know a person, use *conocer*
sad—*triste*
safety—*la seguridad*
safety valve—*la válvula de seguridad*
sal, la—salt
sala de ordeño, la—milking parlor
saladero, el—salt block, salt lick
sale—*la venta*

salegar, la—salt block, salt lick
salida, la—exit
salir—to leave, to go out
salt—*la sal*
salt lick, salt block—*la salegar, el saladero*
saltamontes, el—grasshopper
salud, la—health
saludos, los—greetings
salvado, el—bran
same—*mismo, misma*
sangre, la—blood
Saturday—*el sábado*
scale—*la báscula*
school—*la escuela*
science—*la ciencia*
scraper—*el raspador*
scratched—*raspado, raspada*
scrotum—*el escroto*
season—*el celo;* in season—*en celo*
seco, seca—dry
security—*la seguridad*
sedum—*la hierba callera*
see—*ver*
see ya, be seein' ya—*nos vemos*
seed—*la semilla, el grano*
seem—*parecer;* it seems to me that—*me parece que*
segadora, la—hay swather
seguir (i, i)—to follow, to go straight ahead, to keep going
seguridad, la—security, safety
seguro, el—insurance
seguro, segura—sure; *no estoy seguro/a*—I'm not sure
seguro social, el—Social Security
sell—*vender*
seller—*el vendedor* (male), *la vendedora* (female)
semana, la—week; *semana pasada*—last week
semen—*el semen*
semen, el—semen

semilla, la—seed
seminal vesicle—*la vesícula seminal*
sémola, la—grits, semolina
semolina—*la sémola*
send—*enviar*
sense, to feel—*sentir*
sentir (ie, i)—to feel, to sense; *¿sintió eso?*—did you hear that?
separador, el—separator
separador de estiércol, el—manure separator
separar—to separate
separate—*separar*
separator—*el separador;* milk separator—*la descremadora*
September—*septiembre*
septiembre—September
ser—to be; use with innate characteristics, such as physical appearance or personality
serious, close to death—*grave*
serve—*servir (i, i)*
servir (i, i)—to serve
sexado de embriones, el—embryo sexing
sex—*el sexo*
sexo, el—sex
shade—*la sombra*
shear—*esquilar*
shearing clippers—*la esquiladora*
shearing facilities—*las instalaciones de esquilar*
shearing shed—*la muda*
sheep—*la oveja; el carnero* (ram), *la oveja, la oveja hembra* (ewe)
sheep fold—*el redil*
sheep foot trimmers—*el cortapezuñas*
sheep ranch—*el rancho ovejero*
sheepskin—*el vellón*
shepherd—*el pastor* (male), *la pastora* (female)

shoat (feeder pig)—*el lechón; el cerdo destetado*
shoot (a gun)—*disparar*
short (in length)—*corto, corta*
shovel—*la pala*
show—*mostrar (ue)*
sick—*enfermo, enferma*
sickness—*la enfermedad*
siempre—always
sifón, el—siphon
signature—*la firma*
silage—*el ensilaje*
silo—*el silo*
silo, el—silo
silo con elevador, el—grain elevator
simpático, simpática—nice (used only with humans, not with things or animals)
sin—without; *sin falta*—without fail
sincronización del estro, la—synchronization of estrus
single, unmarried—*soltero, soltera*
siphon—*el sifón*
sistema de ordeño, el—milking system
sistema de piso rasurado, el—slotted floor system
sistema de reproducción, el—breeding system
sister—*la hermana*
skin—*la piel;* sheepskin—*el vellón*
sleep—*dormir (ue, u)*
slotted floor system—*el sistema de piso rasurado*
slowly—*despacio*
small—*pequeño, pequeña; chico, chica*
small intestine—*el intestino delgado*
snake—*la culebra*
snow (verb)—*nevar*
so—*tan;* so difficult—*tan difícil*

so much—*tanto*
so that—*para*
soap—*el jabón* (often spelled *javón*)
sobrevivir—to survive
sobrina, la—niece
sobrino, el—nephew
socia, la—member (of a club)
    (female)
Social Security—*el seguro social*
socio, el—member (of a club) (male)
¡socorro!—help!
soga, la—rope
soil—*el suelo*
sol, el—sun; *hace sol*—it's sunny
soltero, soltera—single, unmarried
sombra, la—shade
someone—*alguien*
sometimes—*a veces*
son—*el hijo*
sonda de ultrasonido, la—
    ultrasonic probe
soon—*pronto*
sorghum—*el sorgo*
sorghum silage—*el ensilado de
    sorgo*
sorgo, el—sorghum
sorry, I'm sorry—*lo siento*
sorting chute—*la manga
    separadora*
sorting pen—*el corral separador*
south—*el sur*
sow—*la cerda, el vientre*
    (female pig)
Spanish language—*el español*
speak—*hablar*
Specific Pathogen-Free (SPF)
    Program—*el programa libre
    de patógenos específicos*
sperm—*el esperma*
spermatozoid—*el espermatozoide*
spirited—*fogoso, fogosa*
spray—*rociar*
sprayer—*el rociador*

spread—*esparcir*
spreader—*la esparcidora*
spring heifer—*la vaquilla a parto*
squeeze chute—*la prensa, la trampa*
stable—*el establo*
stabled—*estabulado, estabulada*
stall—*el pesebre*
starch—*el almidón*
steady (calm)—*tranquillo, tranquilla*
steer—*el torete, el novillo*
sterilize—*esterilizar*
sterilized—*esterilizado,
    esterilizada*
still—*todavía*
sting—*picar* (snakes and insects)
stomach—*el estómago*
storm—*la tormenta;*
    thunderstorm—*el aguacero*
straw—*la paja; la pajilla*
    (used in reproduction)
straw litter—*la cama*
stubble—*el rastrojo*
stuck (to get stuck in)—*atascar*
subasta, la—auction
subir—to go up; to board (a
    vehicle)
substance—*la sustancia*
suceder—to happen, to occur
Sudan grass—*el pasto Sudán*
suelo, el—soil; floor
sufficient—*suficiente*
suficiente—sufficient, enough
    (quantity)
sugar—*el azúcar*
sugerir (ie, i)—to suggest
suggest—*sugerir (ie, i)*
sun—*el sol;* it's sunny—*hace sol*
Sunday—*el domingo*
suplemento, el—supplement
supplement—*el suplemento*
sur, el—*south*
sure—*seguro, segura;* I'm not
    sure—*no estoy seguro/a*

survive—*sobrevivir*
sustancia—substance
swallow—*tragar*
swine—*el ganado porcino, los
cerdos*
swine industry—*la industria
porcina*
synchronization of estrus—*la
sincronización del estro*

T

table—*la mesa*
tail docking—*el descolado*
take care of—*cuidar de*
taller, el—workshop
también—also, too
tame—*manso, mansa*
tan—so; *tan difícil*—so difficult
tangle, to get tangled—*embrollar*
tangled—*embrollado, embrollada*
tank—*el tanque*
tanque, el—tank
tanque de nitrógeno líquido, el—
liquid nitrogen tank
tanto—so much; as much; that much
tarde—late
tarde, la—afternoon (goes on until
seven or eight in the evening)
task—*el quehacer*
tattoo—*tatuar* (verb); *el tatuaje*
(noun)
tatuaje, el—tattooing
tatuar—to tattoo
teat—*la teta, el pezón*
teat cup—*la pezonera*
tela metálica, la—wire mesh
teléfono, el—telephone
telephone—*el teléfono*
tell—*decir;* tell a story—*contar (ue)*
temprano—early
tener—to have, to own; *tener
que*—have to
terminar—to finish, to end

ternera, la—calf (female)
ternero, el—calf (male)
test—*la prueba, el examen*
testicle—*el testículo*
testículo, el—testicle
teta, la—teat
thank God—*gracias a dios*
thank you—*gracias;* thank you
very much—*muchas gracias*
that—*que* (connecting word); *ese,
esa, eso*—that (over there)
that much—*tanto*
there—*allí, allá*
there is, there are—*hay*
thiamin—*la tiamina*
think—*creer* (to have an opinion);
pensar—to contemplate
this—*este, esta, esto*
thorax—*el tórax*
thunder—*el trueno*
thundershower—*el aguacero*
thunderstorm—*el aguacero;
la tormenta*
Thursday—*el jueves*
thus—*así*
tiamina, la—thiamin
tiempo, el—time; weather
tía, la—aunt
tick—*la garrapata*
time—*el tiempo* (clock time);
la vez (instances); three
times—*tres veces*
tío, el—uncle
tire—*la llanta* (on a vehicle)
tired—*cansado, cansada*
to—*a;* when *a* is next to *el,*
they combine to form *al*
toalla, la—towel
toasted—*tostado, tostada*
todavía—still; yet
today—*hoy*
todo, toda—all, all of
toenail—*uña*

tomorrow—*mañana*
too, also—*también*
too much—*demasiado*
tórax, el—thorax
torete, el—steer
tormenta, la—storm
toro, el—bull
torta, la—cake
torta de algodón, la—cottonseed cake
torta oleaginosa, la—oil cake
toser—to cough
tostado, tostada—toasted
tournament—*la competición*
towel—*la toalla*
toxic—*tóxico, tóxica*
tóxico, tóxica—toxic
toxin—*la toxina*
toxina, la—toxin
trabajador, el—worker (male)
trabajadora, la—worker (female)
trabajar—to work
trabajo, el—work
tracto alimenticio, el—alimentary tract
tracto digestivo, el—digestive tract
tractor—*el tractor*
tractor, el—tractor
traer—to bring
tragar—to swallow
trailer—el remolque
trampa, la—squeeze chute
trampa ajustable, la—lockup; cage chute; cage crate
tranquilo, tranquila—calm, steady
transferencia de embriones, la—embryo transfer
trébol, el—clover
tremendo, tremenda—tremendous, awful
tremendous—*tremendo, tremenda*
trinchete, el—fork, pitchfork

triste—sad
triturado, triturada—crushed
troca, la—truck (term used in the United States)
tropical—*tropical*
tropical—tropical
truck—*el camión; la troca* (U.S. slang); pickup truck—*la camioneta*
trueno, el—thunder
tube—*el tubo*
tubo, el—pipe, tube
Tuesday—*el martes*
tuna, la—prickly pear cactus
turkey—*el pavo* (male), *la pava* (female); *el guajolote* (in Mexico)

U

ubre, la—udder
udder—*la ubre*
ugly—*feo, fea*
ulcer—*la úlcera*
úlcera, la—ulcer
últimamente—recently; lately
ultrasonic probe—*la sonda de ultrasonido*
umbilical cord care—*el cuidado del cordón umbilical*
uncle—*el tío*
understand—*entender (ie), comprender*
ungüento, el—ointment
único, única—only, one and only
unidad, la—unit
unidad de crecimiento-finalización, la—growing-finishing unit
unidad de destete—weaning unit
unit—*la unidad*
unload—*descargar*
until—*hasta*
uña, la—toenail, nail

urea—*la urea*
urea, la—urea
usar—to use
use—*usar* (verb); *el uso* (noun)
uso, el—use
útero, el—uterus
uterus—*el útero*

V

vaca, la—cow
vaca lechera, la—milk cow
vaca seca, la—dry cow
vacaciones, las—vacation
vacation—*las vacaciones*
vaccine—*la vacuna*
vacuna, la—vaccine
vagina—*la vagina*
vagina, la—vagina
valor nutritivo, el—nutritional
  value
valve—*la válvula*
válvula, la—valve
válvula de escape, la—escape valve
válvula de seguridad, la—
  safety valve
vaquera, la—cowgirl, cow woman
vaquero, el—cowboy, cowman
vaquilla, la—heifer
vaquilla a parto, la—spring heifer
vecina, la—neighbor (female)
vecino, el—neighbor (male)
vehicle—*el vehículo*
vehículo, el—vehicle; carrier
vellón, el—fleece; sheepskin
vendaje, el—bandage
vendar—to bandage
vendedor, el—seller (male)
vendedora, la—seller (female)
vender—to sell
venir—to come
venta, la—sale (of goods)
ver—to see; *nos vemos*—see ya,
  be seein' ya

verraco, el—male pig, boar;
  often spelled *berraco*
very—*muy;* very well—*muy bien*
vesícula, la—bladder
vesícula biliar, la—gallbladder
vesícula seminal, la—seminal
  vesicle
vetch—*la veza*
veterinaria, la—veterinarian
  (female)
veterinarian—*el veterinario,
  la veterinaria*
veterinario, el—veterinarian
  (male)
vez, la—time (instance); *a
  veces*—sometimes; *otra vez*—
  again; *tres veces*—three times
veza, la—vetch
vida, la—life
viejo, vieja—old
viento, el—wind; *hace viento*—
  it's windy
vientre, el—female pig
viernes, el—Friday
virus—*el virus*
virus, el—virus
vitamin—*la vitamina*
vitamina, la—vitamin
viuda, la—widow
viudo, el—widower
vivir—to live
volver (ue)—to return,
  to come back
vulva—*la vulva*
vulva, la—vulva

W

wait for—*esperar*
wake up—*amanecer*
walk—*andar, caminar*
wallow—*el revolcadero*
want—*querer (ie)*
wash—*lavar*

watch—*mirar*
watch out!—*¡cuidado!*
watch out for—*cuidar de*
water—*el agua*
water hose—*la manguera*
water trough—*el bebedero*
water well—*el pozo*
wean—*destetar*
weaned—*destetado, destetada*
weaning unit—*la unidad de destete*
weather—*el tiempo, el clima*
Wednesday—*el miércoles*
week—*la semana*
weekend—*el fin de semana*
weigh—*pesar*
weighing crate—*la báscula*
weight—*el peso*
welcome—*bienvenido, bienvenida;* you're welcome—*de nada, no hay de qué*
well—*bien*
well done—*bien hecho*
west—*el oeste*
what?—*¿qué?;* what did you say?—*¿cómo?; ¿mande?* (Mexico)
wheelbarrow—*la carretilla*
when—*cuando;* when?—*¿cuándo?*
where—*donde;* where?—*¿dónde?;* to where?—*¿adónde?*
which—*qué;* Which?—*¿Qué?* or *cuál, ¿Cuál?*
white—*blanco, blanca*
who—*quien;* who?—*¿quién?*
widow—*la viuda*
widower—*el viudo*
wife—*la esposa*
wind—*el viento;* it's windy today—*hace viento hoy*

wing—*el* or *la ala*
wing badge—*el arete de la ala*
wing tag—*el arete de la ala*
wire—*el hilo, el alambre*
wire mesh—*la tela metálica*
with—*con*
without—*sin*
without fail—*sin falta*
wool—*la lana*
work—*trabajar* (verb); *el trabajo* (noun)
worker—*el obrero* (male), *la obrera* (female); *el trabajador* (male), *la trabajadora* (female)
workshop—*el taller*
worse—*peor*
wound, injury—*la herida*
wrench—*la llave*
write—*escribir*

X

Y

y—and
ya—already; still; yet
year—*el año;* don't confuse this with *el ano* (anus)
yearling—*el añil*
yegua, la—mare
yesterday—*ayer*
yet—*todavía; ya*
yeyuno, el—jejunum
yield—*rendir*
yodo, el—iodine

Z

zanahoria, la—carrot
zinc—*el zinc*
zinc, el—zinc